FEEDING MANAGEMENT OF WILD ANIMALS IN SITU AND ZOO

FEEDING MANAGEMENT OF WILD ANIMALS IN SITU AND ZOO

Nityanand Pathak
B.Sc., B.V.Sc. & A.H., M.V.Sc., Ph.D., FNAVSI,
FANA, FMOBS, MAAVN
President, Pashu Chikitski Poshan Avam Kalyan Samiti
113B, Vatika, Sun City Vistaar, Izatnagar-243122, U.P.

S.K. Saha
B.V.Sc. & AH, M.Sc.(D), Ph.D.
FNAVS, Post Doc (Australia) Post Doc (USA)
Principal Scientist
Animal Nutrition Division
Indian Veterinary Research Institute
Izatnagar-243122, U.P.

SSPH

SATISH SERIAL PUBLISHING HOUSE
403, Express Tower, Commercial Complex
Azadpur, Delhi-110033 (India)
Phone : 011-27672852, Fax : 91-11-27672046
e-mail : info@satishserial.com, hkjain1975@yahoo.com
Website : www.satishserial.com

Published by :

SATISH SERIAL PUBLISHING HOUSE
403, Express Tower, Commercial Complex, Azadpur, Delhi-110033 (INDIA)
Phone : 011-27672852 Fax : 91-11-27672046
E-mail : info@satishserial.com, hkjain1975@yahoo.com

ISBN 978-93-86200-75-4

Composed, Designed & Printed in India

Preface

The course number VMD012 includes zoo/wild animals breeding, nutrition, management and health care and completed only in 2 (1+1) credit hours of semester IX in the part of Bachelor of Veterinary Science and Animal Husbandry (B.V.Sc. & A.H.) of the Indian Universities. There is probably no concise text book on the feeding of zoo/wild animals of variable food preference, feeding behaviour and nutritional requirements. About three decades ago, I proposed a course on the feeding of wild animals in the course content of Animal Nutrition of the Indian Veterinary Research Institute (Deemed University), Izatnagar. The faculty members faced difficulties in teaching. Initial load was more on me because course was suggested and composed by me. In order to gather teaching materials I organized a summer Institute entitled, "Nutrition and Feeding of Wild Herbivorous Mammals in Captivity" under the annual faculty refresher programme of the Indian Council of Agricultural Research, New Delhi. The lectures were edited by author and co-workers Drs. D.N. Kamra, A.K. Garg and N. Agarwal. This was followed by more elaborate short course during 1999-2000 by Dr. D.N. Kamra, N. Agarwal, L.C. Chaudhary and N.N. Pathak. In 2008, a more expanded course entitled, "Emerging Trends in Nutrition of Wild and Zoo Animals" was compiled by Dr. S.K. Saha, A. Das, N. Dutt, L.C. Chaudhary and K. Sharma. These three compendia of a summer school of ICAR and two of CAS/CAFT of Animal Nutrition Division, Indian Veterinary Research Institute, Izatnagar provide satisfactory informations on the nutrition and feeding of several wild mammalian and few other animals but still many important aspects are not included.

A need was felt for a comprehensive text book on the feeding of zoo and wild animals. It took long time of about 5 years for the preparation of outline and text for the course of veterinary graduates of Indian Universities. My association in a research project on wild animal feeding and management in Wildlife National Park, Dudhwa from 1985-90 and visits to other wild life sanctuaries in India, jungle safari, Mikumi in Tanzania and several zoos in India and other countries was useful in the composition of this book. However, there is enough scope for the elaboration of this course as an independent course of 3 (2+1) credit hours of a semester.

The pleasant environment provided by grand children Ananya, Anuvrat, Atharva, Anavartika and Akshita directly and Anshuman, Aadya and Amulya remotely had helped a lot. The inspiring force is Sushila (March 11, 1967 to March 4, 2004) who spared me from domestic responsibilities and social obligations. Special thanks to Dr. S.K. Saha for keen interest in publication and Padmashini Pathak for proof reading.

Nityanand Pathak

Contents

1

Introduction

Introduction

Life is the most precious gift of Almighty. Through the process of progressive evolution, unicellular life evolved to large number of multicellular creatures distributed on the earth. The life can be described in different ways on the basis of cellular organization as prokaryotes and eucaryotes represented by micro-organisms, flora and fauna. This book is limited to the feeding of wild animals represented mainly by the mammals, reptiles and avian species. The subject is vast and actual scientific informations on the feeding of most of the wild animal species.

The scope of food selection for optimum nutrients supply has decreased significantly due to continuous shrinking of forests, pollution of environment, decrease of natural wetlands and infestation of humans in deep forests and hilly regions causing extensive deforestation. The emission of polluted fumes and drainage of industrial effluents and municipal garbage into the rivers, streams and lakes have significant detrimental effects on the wild fauna. Now many species are either extinct or migrated away from their earlier habitats. Gangentic dolphins (Soos) was quite common in the large rivers like Ganga, Ghaghara, Gandak and others but now they are rarely spotted. The common wild animals of human habitation like Blackbuck, Neelgai and spotted deer and nocturnal animals like jackals, foxes, mongooses and wolves have disappeared from many parts. Today children from the villages also have not heard the howling of jackals and wolves. The common sparrow and other birds nesting in the huts, houses and trees have also disappeared from the large area of human habitation. Similar is the situation of several wild animals commonly living in co-existence with the humans. In conclusion it can be said that threat to wild animals is more from the human socio-cultural development requiring continuous industrial growth.

Existence of many important water sources I now threatened due to unethical human activities. Serious fall in biological oxygen demand (BOD) of rivers due to drainage of municipal garbage and industrial effluents is responsible for the drastic fall in number like turtles in Yamuna river at Mathura and dolphins in the Ganga and Saryu rivers.

The prevailing detrimental activities threatening wildlife have compelled for taking sustainable measures for the conservation of wildlife.

Measures Taken for the Conservation of Wildlife

Some of the important measures taken for the conservation of the wild life can be listed as follows:

1. Ear-marking of reserve forests: This is useful for the conservation of wild plants and animals in situ.
2. Ear-marking of forests as National Wildlife parks, sanctuaries and reserves, etc.
3. Ear-marking of forests as National Wildlife parks, sanctuaries and reserves, etc.
4. Establishment of zoological parks, zoo and zoo Gardens for the protection and conservation of wild animals, lesser known animals and exotic animals, etc.
5. Establishment of bird sanctuaries and protection of water sources used for seasonal habitation by the migratory birds.

Large number of different species of birds including Siberian cranes visit across the Himalaya to their winter habitats in Bharat. Some of these are Kevaladeva Bird Sanctuary, Bharatpur, Surabh tal in Ballia, Ramgarh tal in Gorakhpur, Gudar tal in Jithpur, Kaula jheel in Mathura, Chilka lake in Odisha and many others.

Water streams, ponds, tanks and rivers in deep forests and difficult hilly terrains are preferred by most of the migratory birds. These water sources are relatively less polluted and danger of human predators in little. Human habitants of forests normally hunt few animals/birds for their kitchen from the abundant species. Most of them provide protection to rate and threatened species. However, detrimental activities are also supported by a few *vanvasi* lured by the professional poachers like Chand of Uttrakhand.

Some Important Causes of Poaching

1. Hunting for food: The common animals hunted for food are deer, antelopes, wild boar, hare and different avian species.
2. Hunting for ethnic medicine: The most threatened species are lion, tigers, tusker, elephants and other large cats, wild canines, rhinoceros, crocodile, many avian species and others.

3. Hunted for hide, horns, antlers, feathers and other organs: These are used as trophy, decoration items and ornaments, etc.
4. Reptiles: These are hunted for venom, skin and organs for ethnic medicine, skin and other parts.
5. Feather collection: Some beautiful birds are killed for their valuable feathers. Flesh of such birds is a secondary product. Some examples are peacock, pheasants and ratites like ostrich, rhea, emu and kiwi, etc.
6. For the protection of human and domestic animals: For the families in the periphery of jungle wild canines are big threat. Wolves, hyena and jackals often lift infants, kids, lambs, poultry and even young calves. Some times a pack of wolves and jackals kill human adults and animals straying near the jungle.

Why Attention for Nutrition and Feeding of Wild Animals in Situ

The human intervention in forest management is changing the ecology. The natural water sources running across the forests are mostly polluted by municipal and industrial draining during their course. These have disturbed the herbage composition. Many plant species are vanishing due to which nutritional imbalances are appearing in the wild animals of different regions. These changes need the attention of wild animal managers. For the correction of nutritional imbalances, services of Animal Nutritionists are required. However, in the syllabi of veterinary sciences there is little for the graduates. The veterinarians of the forest and zoo apply their knowledge studied for the domestic animals. The person in zoo mostly follows the empirical menu with some modifications. So far, there is no comprehensive post graduate specialized course or training for the wild animals nutrition and feeding. Author introduced the course on the feeding of wild and zoo animals and also organized a summer course on the feeding of wild herbivorous animals under the annual programmes of the Indian Council of Agricultural Research. This was followed by further courses of the Centre of Advance Studies (CAS) in Animal Nutrition at the Indian Veterinary Research Institute, Izatnagar.

Publication of Summer Course and Courses Organized by CAS and CAFT, Animal Nutrition Division, Indian Veterinary Research Institute, Izatnagar

The following short courses organized by the author and his associates are the part of the instruction and teaching materials for the courses on wildlife feeding at the Veterinary Colleges of the Indian Universities.

1. Pathak, N.N., Kamra, D.N., Garg, A.K. and Agarwal, N. 1996. Nutrition and feeding of wild herbivorous mammals in captivity. Centre of Advance Studies in Animal Nutrition, Indian Veterinary Research Institute (Lectures of Summer School of the Indian Council of Agricultural Research, New Delhi).
2. Kamra, D.N., Agarwal, N., Chaudhary, L.C., Pathak N.N., Garg, A.K. and Sastry, V.R.B. 1999-2000. Nutrition and feeding of wild mammals. Compendium of Centre of Advance Studies in Animal Nutrition, Indian Veterinary Research Institute, Izatnagar.
3. Saha, S.K., Das, A., Dutta, N., Chaudhary, L.C. and Sharma, K. 2008. Emerging trends in nutrition of wild and zoo animals. Compendium of Centre of Advance Studies in Animal Nutrition, Indian Veterinary Research Institute, Izatnagar.

These publications contain valuable information on the nutrition and feeding of wild and zoo animals, but these publications lack the organization pattern of a text book. These publications have some basic aspects included in the course VMD 512. This course is also primitive and requires adequate contents for the optimum feeding of captive animals housed in the limited space of zoos. Indian zoos and wild life reserve forests are mostly managed by the forest departments, which basically utilized the services of veterinarians for management but access of researchers was almost prohibited. Veterinarians also had little interest due to opportunities and indifferent behaviour of the personnel of Indian Forest Service before it was opened for the veterinary graduates.

Need of Nutrition Research on the Wild and Zoo Animals

Due to increasing intervention of human in the forest and wild animals management and increasing environment pollution, the composition of plant species is changing. Commercial forestry has eliminated many edible herbages from many forests. This has adversely affected the nutrition of wild herbivorous animals due to decreased scope of selective feeding. Organized line plantation of valuable timber trees, number and cover of natural bushes, grasses, herbs, creepers and climbers, etc. has significantly decreased. This change in herbage composition along with the shrinking forest area has considerably disturbed the food resources. This has increased trespassing of wild herbivores in the cultivated fields in the periphery of the forest. These animals are frequently followed by the carnivorous animals. Incidence of animal and human predation is increasing in the periphery of forests. Sometimes wild large cats like tigers and leopard, and canines like hyenas and wolves, etc. enter in human habitations far away from the forests and create fear among the people.

Classification of Wild Mammals on the Basis of Food Preference

The wild animals require feeding intervention can be classified into the following classes:

1. Mammals: The mammals are further divided into the following sub-groups:

   1.1. Herbivorous animals: These animals thrive exclusively on eating different kinds of plants. The diets include whole plants, leaves, bark, inflorescence, fruits and roots. On the basis of higher proportion of some components of the plants, the herbivores are further divided as follows :

   1.1.1. Folivorous: The diet of this group contain more than 50% leaves of total intake. A few wild animal species eat the leaves of only few plant species. Koala eats leaves of eucalyptus only.

   1.1.2. Flourivorous: These species eat preferably flowers.

   1.1.3. Frugivorous: These animals prefer to eat fruits of different plants. Fruits are normally eaten on the onset of ripening but raw fruits are also eaten during scarcity.

   1.1.4. Frugivorous : These animals like to eat different species of mushrooms emerging from the ground and growing on the decaying wood and grasses in different season. Wild mushrooms grow more during the wet season. The soil of termite mount and burrows of ants provide nutritious soil for the growth of many mushroom species.

1.1.5. Nectervorous : Some wild animals only lick the nectar present at the base of flowers. In some plants like Kaner, it is secreted as sweet white sap but its large intake may be fatal due to presence of toxin.

1.1.6. Melevorous: Some wild animals specially the bear is crazy for the honey and climbs on the trees for honey eating.

1.2. Carnivorous mammals : All mammals eating more than 50% foods of animal flesh. These animals are further classified on the basis of flesh preferably eaten by the carnivorous animals into the following sub-groups:

1.2.1. Predators : These animals in wild predate preferably wild herbivores. Feline, canine and other carnivores kill deer, antelope, zebra, giraffe, hare, rabbit, rats and others. The other species predated include wild buffaloes and rarely elephant calves. Domestic animals are predated by wild carnivores straying out of the forest.

1.2.2. Scavengers : These are mostly foxes and disabled members of other carnivores.

1.2.3. Piscivorous mammals : Dolphins and whales are aquatic animals feeding on fishes and other aquatic animals. They also eat small quantity of algae and other aquatic herbages.

1.2.4. Amphibious herbivorous mammals : Some mammals live in water but graze grasses on the ground. These are rhinoceros, swamp buffalo and hippopotamus, etc.

1.2.5. Amphibious piscivorous mammals : These animals live in water for longer hours of the day and eat fishes, frogs, crabs, lobsters, etc.

1.3. Omnivorous mammals : The diets of such mammals include forages, fallen grains, fruits and kernels, etc. These animals also eat left over flesh, decaying carcass and sometimes kill small animals like rat, mouse, hare and rabbits, etc.

Feeding Time of the Mammals

A hungry animal eats any time on the availability of feeds but as per natural adaptation they are (i) diurnal and (ii) nocturnal.

i) Diurnal feeding : Most of the large herbivores graze/browse during the comfortable hours of the day light. In cold season they feed during mid day and during warm months they feed at dawn and dusk.

ii) Nocturnal feeding : Some animals like pygmy pig, porcupine, moles and some canine species feed during the night.

Feeding Strata of the Herbivorous Mammals

The herbivorous animals are grouped on the basis of feeding strata on natural herbages into the following classes:

1. Ground level feeder or grazers : These species feed on grasses and rarely eat shrubs or tree leaves. These are wild buffalo, wild sheep, yak, gaur and feral cattle.
2. Middle level feeders : These animals consume substantial amount of succulent barks in addition to grazing and browsing on shrubs and short trees. These include deer, antelopes and mithun.
3. Top feeders : The tall animals with long neck like camels and giraffe preferably browse on the tree leaves. This is convenient for the long neck. Wild elephants are proboscis for apprehension and engulfing. Most species of primates, squirrels and koala, etc. are selective top feeders.
4. Aquatic and swamp feeders : Mammals living most of the time in water eat aquatic plants and aquatic animals as per their food preference.
   a) Aquatic herbivores : The animals of swamp and water like rhinoceros and buffaloes eat aquatic herbages and other plants of wet land. Chilka buffalo of Odisha have been evolved to feed on the submerged plants and emerge full mouth bite for chewing and swallowing.
   b) Aquatic carnivores : Aquatic mammals are found in the fresh water and ocean. They eat fishes, amphibians and crustaceans. The true stomach of grey whale is preceded by three large compartments harbouring micro-organisms for digestion as observed in the ruminants.

Frugivorous and Herbivorous Relationship for Food Sharing in Wild

Several examples of co-existence of wild animal species have been recorded form the wild life reserve forests. The most common example is the relationship of monkeys and small ruminants of deer and antelope groups in the tropical forests. The event is more common during the dry season. The grasses mature but trees carry plant fruits and green leaves. The monkeys move from branch to branch for eating fruit. In this process good amount of fruits fall and also partly eaten or bitter fruits of different stages of maturity are thrown down. The monkeys also pluck and throw the twigs with green leaves. These are eaten by the animals clustering beneath the tree. On close observations for few days one can observe the quadruped herbivores demanding foods from the monkeys on the trees. This situation is more common beneath the jamum (*Euglena jambolina*), banyan tree (*Ficus bergalensis*), gular tee (*Fiscus glomerata*) and many others. Some monkeys tease the begging animals and throw fruits here and there or holding in hand post to throw but delay throwing and enjoy the running of animals beneath the tree for foods. The act is friendly and example of co-operation in hard jungle life.

Similarly, frugivorous birds like parrots, bulbul and many others throw down large amount of immature and mature fruits, flowers and leaves, which are eaten by small ruminants clustering beneath the fruit trees. Some forests also contain mango trees of small variety having relatively larger kernel and little pulp. The pulp of ripen fruits is eaten by monkeys, squirrel and birds and stones and peels are thrown on the ground to be eaten by the antelopes, deer and other animals.

Classification of Reptiles on the Basis of Food Preference

Almost all reptiles are carnivorous and their food preference has been evolved on the available prey in the habitations. The size of animals and habitats significantly influence the feeding behaviours. The reptiles range from small size insectivorous like house lizards to large size crocodiles, pythons and anaconda capable of predating large herbivorous beats like buffalo, giraffe, zebra, deer and antelope, etc. Some reptiles have preference for specific foods and can be identified accordingly.

1. Large mammals killers like crocodiles, pythons, anaconda and some large lizard.
2. Small animal eaters predating kids, lambs, mouse, rat, hare and rabbits, etc.
3. Ovivorous : Some tree snakes develop liking for eggs. They eat the eggs of birds and also the chicks.
4. Insectivorous : These are small reptiles like house lizards.
5. Scavengers : They feed on dead carcasses and left over of other Carnivores.
6. Piscivorous : Aquatic reptiles predate fishes, crabs, lobsters, snails and amphibians.

Classification of Avian Species on the Basis of Food Preference

Like mammals avian species can be classified as herbivorous, omnivorous and carnivorous. Most of the species are omnivorous and their diets include grains, tender leaves, insects, larvae and pupae.

1. Herbivorous birds : Greater proportion of goods are grains, fruits, flowers, leaves, etc. some of the examples are parrot, pigeon, sparrow, bulbul and myna, etc. all ratites are herbivores.
2. Carnivores
   i) Cadover eaters including bulchers, owl, hawks, eagle and crow, etc.
   ii) Insectivorous are mostly small birds like sparrow, etc.
   iii) Piscivorous eat small fishes, spawn, fingerlings, tadpole, amphibians and crustaceans, etc.
   iv) Predators : These birds predate small mammals, amphibians, reptiles and chicks, etc. Common predator are kite, eagle, hawks, owl and crow, etc.
3. Melevorous : Some wild birds addicted for the nectar and honey possess very long beaks slightly curved at the tip for sucking nectar at the base of flowers.
4. Frugivorous : Some avian species like red vent and yellow vent bulbuls and probably parrots are unable to synthesize vitamin C

and need dietary supplementation. These birds eat guava and other citrus fruits for the supply of vitamin C.

5. Omnivorous : Large species of birds are omnivorous and more than half of the diets is mostly grains, seeds, kernels an tender leaves. Non-herbaceous foods are insects, larvae, pupae, earthworms and tiny animals. Some birds like peacock also eat small snakes. Some large kites lift small turtles quite high in the sky and then leave to fall on the hard rock. The hard shield of the turtle splits into pieces and flesh is eaten by the kite.

Crows are very notorious and they take long time for killing a frog, mice and other small animals. Crows enjoy the painful crying of their preys.

Reasons for the Establishment of Zoo

Following are the main reasons of establishment of zoo or zoological gardens in an area of a state or country :

1. Conservation of the endangered wild animal species of the state.
2. Display of wild animal species in a well managed initiated wild environment in the safe enclosures of a zoological garden.
3. Housing of the wild and uncommon species of the other states of the country.
4. Housing and display of wild animals translocated from the other countries.
5. To provide opportunity to local public to see wild animal species. It is normally difficult for every citizen to see the wild animals, their behaviour and habitat. Zoos provide opportunity to all class of people, specially to economically weaker section unable to save money for visits of wildlife sanctuaries and parks, etc.
6. Source of education for the students of biological sciences and ecology. Students get opportunity to see live specimens of good number of mammals, reptiles and avian species at one place freely roaming inside the safe enclosures.
7. Training of the veterinary graduates for approaching, handling, restrain, clinical examination, drug administration, feeding and management. Earlier it was a casual approach of teaching but in revised syllabus specific course on wild and zoo animals has been introduced in the veterinary courses of the Indian Universities.

8. Place of relaxation after busy schedule for a week, fortnight, month or longer interval. Zoological gardens containing parts with blossoming flowers and beds of green grass carpet. There may be fountains also.

Site Selection for the Establishment of a Zoo

Zoo is a place for housing the wild and uncommon animals of highly variable behaviour in a campus managed by humans specialized for the job. The size of a zoo depends on the available resources. A zoo is normally established in the region of big cities and towns, where life is very busy and most of the residents do not get opportunity to visit jungle safari and see rate wild animals.

Points to be Considered Before the Establishment of a Zoo

Following points should be kept in mind during site selection for the establishment of a zoo:

1. Feasibility of continuity of the zoo.
2. Type of land : Undulating land comprising of plains and bullocks is considered good for a zoo.
3. The land should preferably possess a sub-surface hard plate for minimum loss of water through percolation from the artificial lakes for aquatic animals.
4. Agro-climatic conditions should be suitable for growing different kinds of trees, shrubs and creepers for providing protection from solar exposure, reducing ambient temperature, purification of air and wind breaking, etc.
5. It should be away from the high ways and railway tracks for avoiding continuous noise as far as possible.
6. The site should be reasonably away from the cities, towns, industrial establishments, brick kilns and human habitation.
7. There should not be abattoir, fish ponds, fish markets, meat processing factory and carcass utilization centre at least in 20 km radium of the outer boundary.
8. There should be round the year assured water supply.
9. There should be regular power supply and there should be also arrangement of working generator set with adequate fuel oil.

10. There should be forage farming in the area for the regular supply of fresh green forages throughout the year.
11. Sources of flesh supply for the carnivores should be at reasonable distance.
12. The zoo should be linked by road with the railway station and bus stands and also with the host city/town.
13. There should be reasonably equipped veterinary hospital with indoor patient housing facilities, medicines, appliances and trained staff members.
14. There should not be any construction or other infrastructure at least in 20 km radium of the outer boundary.
15. The height of a very strong outer boundary wall should be 10-15 meters.
16. The outer surface of the boundary wall should be free from any creepers and climbing plants. There should not be tree plantation in a radium of 10 m on either side of the wall.
17. A metallic road of about 3 m width should run along the boundary wall for guarding and service.
18. There should be adequate land at a distance of not less than 3 km for the zoo office, staff residences, stands for motor vehicles and canteen, etc.
19. There must be footbath for every body at the entrance.
20. Feed stores should be inside the zoo but in a separate area opening through separate gate. There should be wide footbath for dipping the wheels of tractors, trolleys, and trucks, etc.
21. There should be properly equipped kitchen for the preparation of soup, slurry and other cooked foods, if zoo is housing species requiring cooked foods.

Precautions in Handling and Feeding

1. All foods must be handled hygienically.
2. Employees for handling and feeding should use sterilized gloves.
3. Food dispensing appliances should be clean and dry.

4. No visitor should be allowed to offer any food.
5. Aggressive, old and weak inmates should not be fed in group.
6. Females in advance pregnancy must be separated from the group at right stage.
7. Spoiled, decaying, foul smelling and moldy foods must not be fed.
8. Weekly fasting (partial or complete) can be followed for the maintenance of good bowel health.
9. Feeding schedule should be followed strictly.
10. Wholesome running drinking water should be available.

Purpose for Wild Animal Conservation in the Forests

The forests are the natural habitat of wild life where animals, plants and other creatures co-exist in the balanced state. Inspite of great difference in food habits and behaviour, herbivores, carnivores and omnivores live together. It will be very difficult task to conserve the large number of wild species in man made environment. The objectives of conservation of wild life (animals, plants and microorganisms) in the natural jungles, hills, wetlands, savannah, deserts, ocean, mountains, arctic and antarctic regions can be listed as follows :

1. Living creatures have been evolved to thrive in co-existence under the conditions of the jungles, wetlands, hills, mountains and deserts, etc.
2. Food resources are available for each species in a characteristic cycle for each geo-climatic condition.
3. Ratio of species is normally maintained by physiological changes in different environment. For example, lush growing edible herbages favour good health and prolific breeding of herbivores. This in continuation provide adequate prey for the carnivores.
4. Management of jungles is less expensive.
5. Natural jungles provide suitable shelter, food and resting place for different species of diverse nature.
6. Natural factors like air, water, light, rains, thunder etc. under diurnal variation maintain balance among the living creatures.

7. In free living condition wild animals are free to make seasonal territory change. This occurs due to drastic change in climate, and scarcity of foodstuffs and water. Seasonal migration is an annual activity of the Siberian birds that migrate mostly to their ancestral destination in the tropical countries.

   Migration of wild animals of African countries in search of food and water can be seen on the television screen. Such programmes are screened by Discovery and other channels of wild life. Territorial trespass among the neighbouring nations is quite common for many species. Movement of elephant clans is almost an annual activity. They move freely in the territory of Bharat, Nepal, Bhutan, Bangladesh and Myanmar.

8. Control of pollution is easier : Human activities causing environmental pollution can be resulted, minimized or even controlled.

9. Unlike conservation in the zoos, arrangements for foods and water supply are normally not required.

Purpose for the Protection of Natural Water Bodies and Wetlands

Perennial water bodies are the habitat of aquatic animals comprising of mammals, reptiles, birds, amphibians and many lower animals. Water bodies and their periphery remain cool due to herbages. These herbages provide foods, shelter and also habitat for many species.

Most of the rivers of Bharat are now polluted due to continuous drainage of industrial effluents and domestic wastes of cities and towns. These have destroyed several aquatic and semi-aquatic species. Restriction on pollution will take long time for controlling the pollution of rivers but it is possible to control the pollution of natural lakes and ponds in the deep forests. However, delay in controlling the pollution of lakes in the jungles of hilly areas. Development of human colonies, resorts and housing for the tourists near such water bodies will spoil the environment. This will reduce the perching of migratory birds. Some of the natural water bodies threatened for the man made pollutions are the natural lakes of Kumaon, Uttar Pradesh, Rajasthan, Chandigarh, Haryana, Odisha and many other states.

If necessary for the economic development human activities may be permitted atleast out of 5 km periphery with the condition of drainage away from the lakes. There should not be industrial activities in the area except the small forest based cottage industries for providing livelihood employment to local artisans.

Periodic Action for the Maintenance of Clean Wholesome Water in Natural Water Bodies

Deposition of decaying fallen leaves, excreta of aquatic animals and eroded soil reduces the depth, water holding capacity and carrying capacity of the aquatic animals and semi-aquatic animals. Therefore, for the maintenance of health natural water bodies, following actions may be taken as per feasibility in the area of water bodies:

1. Removal of silt rich in organic manure, wherever it is possible. The farmers of the accessible area will be happy to take away the valuable silt for the enrichment of their arable lands. This will provide opportunity for increasing organic farming, which will be more remunerative.
2. Introduction of insectivorous aquatic animals, which do not have adverse effect on the existence of aquatic and semi-aquatic wild animals.
3. Cultivation of aquatic plants capable of selective absorption of heavy metals and some harmful chemicals.
4. Periodic attempt for the maintenance of aquatic species ratio in the water bodies.
5. Development of aquatic animals' safari for the generation of resources required for the maintenance of the natural water bodies.

❑❑❑

2

Identification of Domestic Animal Models for the Nutritional Assessment of Wild and Captive Animals

Introduction

All domestic animals have several wild relatives, which are closely related in food preference, feeding behaviours, nutrients utilization and requirements for different physiological functions. The feeds and nutritional requirements of such domesticated animals can be used to meet the nutritional requirements of their wild cousins to greater satisfaction. Wild and captive wild animals belong to mammals, reptiles and aves. These classes possess terrestrial, arborial and aquatic species. A few species of some classes are unable to tolerate the climate to some season and undergo hibernation.

Identification of Domestic Animal Models for the Nutrition of Wild Animals in Captive Conditions

There is a great variation in the shape and size of animals, structure and functions of guts, food preference, feeding behaviour and nutritional requirements of different species of animals. Human, animals and herbage relationship has developed with the evolution of life on the earth. They have both useful and harmful effects on each other. Indeed there are several recorded and not yet recorded relationships among them. Humans are mentally most developed among all the animal due to which they have developed methods for the control and management of even the highly dangerous animals wild large felines (lion, tiger, leopard, cheetah, jaguar, puma, etc), wild canines (wolves, hyena, jackals and dogs, etc), wild pachyderms (elephants and rhinoceros), wild reptiles (snakes, pythons, crocodile, etc) and many other species.

Modern human has high affinity for the nature and wants conservation of all living creatures on the earth in a balanced ecological system. Due to unbalanced growth of humans and other lives, the pressure on food, water and habitats has increased manifolds. This has ultimately turned into conflict among the species for survival. The situation has been further aggravated by the extensive industrial development causing extensive environmental pollution. This prompted mankind for protecting and conserving the life on the earth and also maintaining ecological balance. This has resulted in the global development of wildlife parks, safaris, zoological gardens, botanical gardens, aquarium and reserve forests, etc. earlier zoos and botanical gardens were established by princes and rich people. Later on these were recognized excellent education material for the students of biology, environmental science and ecology.

Nutrition is one of the most important factors for sustaining the normal physiological functions of a living creature. Therefore, it is essential to know the foods and their utilization by the different species of wild animals. It is very difficult for any person to study the nutrition and feeding of the all species of wild animals. Therefore, it is essential to identify a domestic cousin having comparable food preference, feeding and nutrition.

In the absence of a domestic cousin another near relatives have been identified for the selection of feeds/foods and estimating the food and nutritional requirements of the wild animals maintained in captive conditions of the zoological gardens and restricted areas of the wildlife safari and reserves.

For the inmates of the zoological gardens supply of balanced diets is required, whereas for the inmates of wildlife sanctuaries balance among the herbages, herbivores, omnivores and predators is required. Sometimes, supplements of minor nutrients like area specific minerals is also required. In case of natural calamities supply of foods/feeds and water is also required.

Points for the Identification and Selection of Domestic Animal Models

Following factors are generally considered for the selection of domestic animal models for the estimation of food and nutrients requirements of wild animals kept in the zoological gardens:

1. Food preference
2. Diversity in food preference
3. Types of mouth and dentition pattern in different types of animals
4. Types of the digestive systems
5. Feed fermentation vats in the ruminants and non-ruminant animals:
    a) Voluminous rumen in ruminants
    b) Voluminous compartment-1 (C1) in pseudo ruminants (cameloids)

c) Four chambered microbes inhabitating stomach system in colabine monkeys

d) Four chambered microbes inhabitating stomach system in (grey and brown) whales

e) Mid gut microbial digestion in caecum and colon

f) Voluminous caecum for microbial digestion.

g) Provision for caecotrophy and coprophagy.

h) Types of faecal void depicting the moisture absorption capacity and sacculation intensity evident from the shape, size, hardness and amount of faecal pellets.

i) Length of intestine and frequency of excreta void in herbivorous birds.

6. Nursing duration and litter size in the mammalian species.

7. Nutritional cycle of natural herbages of the wildlife parks and minerals in the natural water resources and soils. These informations are useful for the estimation and supply of feed supplements during the scarcity period. This is normally dry summer in the tropics and dry winter in the temperate zone. Seasonal migration is common for the search of food, water, shelter and protection from the predators including humans.

Domestic Animal Models for Herbivorous Mammals

The diets of herbivorous mammals include grasses, herbs, shrubs, trees and aquatic plants. Few species of herbivorous mammals also eat different species of non-toxic algae, lichens, ferns and fungi. Domestic mammals are classified into the following 3 groups on the basis of their structure and functions of the digestive systems:

Ruminants and pseudo ruminants : This is a very large group of herbivorous animals. True ruminants possess very voluminous pregastric chambers for the storage and digestion of herbaceous feeds. The pregastric compartments of the polychambered stomach system are the rumen, reticulum and omasum, and fourth chamber abomasums is the true or glandular stomach. In the pseudo-ruminants (camels and cameloids) the third chamber (equivalent to smasum of true ruminants) is rudimentary.

The first chamber, rumen is the main site for the digestion of fibrous feeds and harbour different species of anaerobic bacteria, archaea, protozoa, fungi and phases for the digestion of lignocellulosic part of the ingested feeds. The population and proportion of different classes of micro-organisms vary considerably among the ruminants and pseudo ruminants and mostly depend on the types of herbages eaten.

Domestic Animal Models for Large Ruminants

Domestic large ruminants are cattle (*Bos indicus* and *Bos taurus*) and Asiatic buffaloes (*Bubalus bubalis*). Two subspecies of domestic Asiatic buffaloes are the dairy type Indian buffalo (*Bubalus bubalis bubalis*) with 2n=50 chromosomes and the Asiatic swamp buffalo (*Bubalus bubalis swampis*)

Food preference of both bovine species is identical and there are non-significant differences in feed intake, digestibility of feeds and nutrients requirement for maintenance. However, nutrients requirement of fattening beef cattle and lactating buffaloes are significantly higher due to higher fat deposition in body and higher fat content in milk, respectively.

The wild bovine species are gaur (*Bos baurus*), Asiatic wild swamp buffalo (*Bubalus arnee*), anoa (*Bubalus depressicornis*) and tamarow or Mindoro buffalo (*Bubalus mindorensis*) in Asia, African wild buffalo (*Syncerus caffer* and *Syncerus nanus*) in Africa, and Bison spp (*Bison bison* and *Bison*) in Europe and Americas. These are close relatives of domestic bovines and can be maintained optimally on the feeds eaten by the domestic bovines. The nutritional requirements for various physiological functions can be applied successfully when applied on the basis of metabolic body weight ($W^{0.75}$) for maintenance, per unit gain in body weight and fat percentage as well as daily milk yield in lactating wild bovines kept in captive conditions of the zoo.

Domestic Animal Models for Small Ruminants

Small ruminants belong to two major groups on the basis of feed preference and feeding behaviours. These are (a) graziers and (b) browsers. These are mostly animals of dry areas (arid and semi-arid) of tropical, sub-tropical and temperate zones. The two main classes are ovines and caprines. The ovines have been evolved as grazing ruminants whereas caprines have been evolved as browsing cum grazing ruminants. The animals of both groups are evolved for thriving in dry areas. They posses long and sacculated large intestine that extends retention time of digesta and provides longer time and more surface area for the absorption of water, minerals particularly electrolytes and some other nutrients. The droppings are pelleted and contain high dry matter percentage, when compared to bovine dung.

Domestic sheep is a suitable model for all species of wild ovines. Domestic goats are suitable models not only for the wild goats but also for the antelopes and most of the cervids (deer) except few evolved in highly specific regions like reindeer, musk deer and swamp deer, etc.

Domestic Animal Models for the True and Pseudoruminants

Camels (Bacterian and Dromedary) and cameloids and llamaids (Llama, Alpaca and Vicuna) obtain greater proportion of nutrition from browsing but vicuna from grazing. The dry matter digestion efficiency of cameloids is about 9-12% higher than the ponies and sheep (Table 2.1). Dietary fibre (cellulose nd hemicellulose) digestion is much higher in cameloids than the ponies and sheep.

Table 2.1 Comparison of digestibility coefficients among camelids, ponies and sheep.

Nutrients	Camelids	Ponies	Sheep
	Experiment 1 (*ad lib* alfalfa hay)		
Dry matter	71.5	64.8	63.8
Crude protein	74.7	66.7	69.7
NDF	60.4	60.1	59.5
ADF	61.0	46.7	
Cellulose	77.6	61.2	64.8
	Experiment 2		
Dry matter	78.5	69.7	71.3
Crude protein	69.2	68.8	63.1
NDF	68.6	45.4	44.7
ADF	38.7	29.3	34.0
Cellulose	47.2	34.5	39.4

Domestic Animal Model for Wild Equines

Zebra and wild asses of India (Runn of Kacch), Africa and central Asia are the wild cousin of domestic equines. Feed preference and nutritional requirements are generally comparable but not similar. Dehydration toleration of Somali donkey is very high and may survive upto 40% water loss. Rehydration is very quick and dehydrated animals regain original body weight within few minutes are drinking water. Domestic pony is a satisfactory model for the assessment of the feed and nutritional requirements of the wild equines kept in captive management.

Domestic Animal Model for Elephants and Rhinoceros

Perhaps there is no domestic animal for use as a model for the nutritional requirements of the elephants and rhinoceros. In natural habitat both species consume large amount of herbages. Browsers are the bulk of elephant diets which include tree leaves as well as branches. The rhinoceros thrives on tall growing coarse grasses of wetlands and also the emerged aquatic grasses. Under free living conditions there is a seasonal. Migration of elephant herds to green forests and water sources. Both the species like wallowing and bathing for several hours.

The diets of captive elephants are formulated on the basis of the diets of domestic (tamed) elephants. Domestication of elephant is quite old in the Indian sub-continent and most of the tropical south-east Asian nations. Different formulae of regional diets are used for the feeding of elephants in the south and south-east Asian countries. The diets of the elephants of the forest department are tall mostly tree fodders, sugarcane and grasses supplements with concentrates. The elephants in temples receive higher proportion of concentrates in ration.

Domestic Animal Models for Wild Lagomorphs

Domestic rabbit is an appropriate model for working out the diets of wild lagomorphs. The diets are predominantly grasses, tubers, roots, fruits and seeds of wild herbages. They also consume cultivated crops in their locality.

Lagomorphs are monogastric herbivores but their digestion processes are somewhat different. A mechanism of digestion of microbial proteins has been evolved by caecotrophy. Caecotrophe is a semi-solid digesta of caecum and contains important metabolites and large number of microorganisms comparable with the ruminal micro-organisms. The caecotrophe is self sucked by the animals during dark hours and redigested in the stomach and small intestine. This process significantly reduce the requirement of dietary digestible protein, energy and almost all vitamins.

Lagomorphs are herbivorous and require adequate fibrous feeds for optimum digestion and the maintenance of gut health. Dietary fibre content below 9% of dry matter and high percentage of starch often develop digestive disorders and sequilae is generally fatal. Some literatures call lagomorphs as pseudoruminants, but camelids are also referred as pseudoruminants. Actually camelids are like true ruminants with 3 or 4 chambered stomach and should be allied humenoids, and the lagomorphs should be called pseudo ruminants.

Domestic Animal Models for Omnivorous Mammals

The omnivorous animals eat variety of foods consisting of food grins, leafy vegetables, fruits, roots, tubers, nuts and grasses. They also eat meat, fish and eggs. The omnivorous animals may be classified into the (i) classical omnivorous animals like primates, swine, hippopotamus and many rodents and (ii) conditioned or adapted omnivorous animals. These are carnivorous animals which adapted omnivorous feeding due to their proximity with human life. Some of the common omnivorous animals are the dogs and cats living in the human colonies. These are neither true domesticated nor true wild animals. These animals receive their foods from casual offerings, garbage, snatching and stealing form the kitchen. Cats frequently hunt rats, caged pet birds, chicken and free living community birds. Street dogs in human habitation are kept controlled by the people but the groups straying in fields, gardens, fallow lands and other areas away from the human habitation become predators and hunt rabbits, hares, fawn and other small animals. Some times large groups of feral dogs also kill small deer species, small antelopes, bovine calves, oats, sheep, kids and lambs.

Some times stray dogs become very dangerous for the humans. Incidence of killing and eating children is often reported. Adult women and weak persons are also predated. Such incidence is more common in areas where carcasses are left open on the ground, thrown in shallow pits or flown in water. This is reversal of feeding behaviour due to increased and easy availability of dead bodies.

Domestic Animal Model for the Common Primates

The diets of omnivorous humans are quite suitable for the primates. They are capable of utilizing raw foods that include water soaked food grains, coarse ground food grains, roots, tubers and fruits. They also eat tender leaves, buds and flowers. The non-vegetarian foods include eggs, milk, meat and some species of fishes. Primates normally do not eat dead and decaying animals. Non-vegetarian foods are not preferred by many primate species.

Domestic Animal Model for Colabine Monkey

Colabine monkey possesses three well formed pregastric chambers that harbour microbial population similar to ruminants for the digestion of fibrous tree leaves. Thus, greater proportion of fodder tree leaves and other succulent forages can be fed with cereals, barns, cakes and fruits.

Domestic Animal Model for Wild Pigs, Hippopotamus and Pygmy Pig

Generally these are herbaceous animals and preferably eat low fibre starchy feeds like succulent roots, tubes, aquatic plants, fruits, berries, seeds, kernels and grasses. These animals also eat seeds and kernels voided in excreta of other animals, flesh of fallen animals and aquatic animals. Domestic pig is a suitable model for the assessment of food and nutritional requirements. Being lethargy maintenance requirement of hippopotamus is less than the pigs.

Domestic Animal Model for Carnivorous Wild Mammals

This is a large group which includes wild mammals, reptiles, avian species and other animals. The diets of carnivorous animals include from insects to large mammals. Almost all species of feline are predators. The wild canines feed on dead bodies and left over of felines but they are also predators. The crocodiles and alligators are predators but also eat dead cadavers. The snakes and pythons are generally predators and most of them swallow entire animal. The selection of prey normally depends on the size of the mouth and flexibility of the alimentary canal. The snakes and pythons are unable to move for many hours after engulfing the prey. Pythons hunt rodents, lagomorphs, antelopes, deer and some time large mammals. Common carnivorous avian species are the vultures, hawk, eagle, kites, crows and owl, etc. aquatic birds and those living on wet lands are predators of fishes, amphibian species and other aquatic animals.

Carnivorous Mammals

Free range and captive wild carnivorous mammals include the following groups :

Feline : Some of the spices of this group are Lion (*Felis leo*), tiger (*Felis tigris*), panther, leopard, cheetah, jaguar, puma, wild cat, civil cat.

Canines : Jackal, hyena, wolves, foxes

Ursids : Bear

Models for the Carnivorous Animals

It is very difficult to find an appropriate model for the carnivorous animals because most of the species are highly dangerous and sensitive. Confinement shock often terminating fatal for many species creates problem in nutritional studies for the preparation of feeding schedule. For the feeding of most of the carnivorous species empirical systems prepared from the experience of hunters and observations in the captive environment are still used. However, pet dogs and cats are used for the nutritional evaluation of flesh and fish based diets.

❑❑❑

3

Foods of Wild and Zoo Animals

Introduction

It is not easy and practical to identify the foods of all animal species on the earth. Almost all animal species are dependent on the organic compounds (carbohydrates, proteins, lipids and vitamins) synthesized and minerals absorbed by the plants from the soil and water sources. Water is the medium for the transportation of nutrients and occurrence of chemical reaction. The source of energy is the sun and gases (carbon dioxide, oxygen, nitrogen and hydrogen) required for the synthesis of organic nutrients are obtained from the environment.

Main Classes of Wild and Rare Animals Normally Kept in Captivity

Due to involvement of large initial cost and the cost of maintenance, it is difficult to establish and maintain big zoos housing large number of specimens of different species of diverse nature, behaviour and food habits. Therefore, in the establishment of a zoo, attempts are made to house such wild nimals, which are normally beyond the reach of common people. The inmates housed in Bhartiya zoos can be classified in different ways as follows:

a) Classes of exotic mammals

The animals for zoos are imported from many other countries. These animals are normally not found in the translocated country. These are mostly rare animals and produce more eagerness in the people for attracting the visitors to zoo. These exotic animals can be placed in the following groups:

1. Exotic herbivorous mammals : Exotic herbivorous mammals imported in the Bhartiya zoos are the giraffe, gnu, African wild buffalo (Synceus sp), Llamas, African elephant, double hump camel, kangaroos, coala, panda and several species of antelopes, cervids, equine, caprine and ovine, etc.
2. Exotic carnivorous mammals : These include different species of big cats (African lion, tiger, puma, cheetah and leopard, etc), canines and ursids, etc.

3. Exotic omnivorous animals : These include rare primates like Gorilla, Chimpanzee, Baboon, many species of monkey and apes, etc.
4. Exotic aquatic mammals : Hippopotamus, dolphins, otters and whales, etc.
5. Exotic arborial mammals : These are mostly selective herbivorous (sometimes omnivorous) animals. These animals spend longer period on trees. Some of the species like to live in caves on the hills and other elevated places.
6. Exotic mammals living in burrows : The mammals of this group spend most hours of day light in the burrows and warrens made underground in the forests and wastelands. Some of mammals of this group include rabbits, jackals, foxes and wolves, etc.

b) Classes of exotic reptiles

1. Exotic lizards : These are insectivorous but large size lizards also hunt small animals.
2. Exotic snakes : These are as usual insectivorous and carnivorous animals.
3. Exotic pythons : These are large size snakes and obtain foods by hunting the animals in their approach.
4. Exotic tortoise : These are found in fresh water and thrive on the aquatic animals.
5. Exotic turtles : These live in saline water and thrive on the flesh and carcass of the animals in the seas and oceans.
6. Exotic crocodiles : Crocodiles are found from fresh water to saline water of different countries. Fresh water crocodiles are always found in the large size water bodies regularly visited by other animals to be hunted for food. The large mouth with rows of strong teeth and strong serrated tail are used for the hunting of even large animals like buffaloes, zebra, antelopes and cervids, etc. In droughts fresh water crocodiles of dried water bodies travel long distance in the direction of newer water sources.

c) Classes of exotic avian species

Avian species basically divided into (a) feathered and (b) featherless (ratite) groups. Although most of the avian species are omnivorous but there are also species preferably eating flesh, while others eat large quantity of grasses.

1. Exotic carnivorous avian species: These birds rarely eat very small quantity of green herbages probably for the supply of carotenes. These birds consume greater proportion of the gut contents of the prey for the supply of vitamins. Some examples are vultures, owls and hawks, etc.
2. Exotic omnivorous avian species: Most of the non-carnivorous avian species extract nutrients from the grains, flowers, tender leaves, nectar, etc. These species consume small quantity of insects, larvae and pupae, etc. Some species also eat tiny mammals and other animals.
3. Exotic aquatic and wetland avian species: These include different wild species of duck, geese, swan, pelcons and herons, etc. These birds eat fishes, amphibians, tadpoles and eggs, etc. They also eat variable quantity of algae, small floating ferns and the aquatic herbages. Some species eat considerable quantity of herbages and considered to possess microbial digestion segments in the large intestine.
4. Exotic ratites (featherless birds): The known domestic, feral and wild species of known ratites are emu, ostrich, rhea and kiwi. Each is represented by several subspecies. Although these are omnivorous species but greater proportion of the diets of most of the ratites is natural herbages. Faster rate of passage (8-12 hours) through the alimentary canal helps quicker nutrients extraction. Microbial digestion occurs in small and large intestine. Coprophagy is extensive in most of the ratites.

d) Classes of indigenous wild animals for zoo

Indigenous wild animals and area specific domestic animals are housed in the zoos for the awareness of people about the animals of different parts of the country. These are also live specimens for education. As in the case of exotic animals, indigenous animals also belong to mammals, reptile and avian species. In a vast nation like Bharat naturally gifted by large number of the mammalian, reptile and avian species, it is difficult to translocate and maintain many species evolved for a highly specific environmental conditions viz. yak on snow covered mountains, camels in dry desert, rhinoceros in swamps and many others.

Sources of Basic Foods

Plants are the basic foods which are capable of synthesizing organic compounds for nutrients supply to animals. The elements and simple gases like oxygen, nitrogen and carbon dioxide are absorbed by the plants and then processed through a series of chemical reactions in the presence of chlorophyll (green pigments) and many enzyme systems. The source of energy is the sun light. The chemical compounds synthesized by the plants for the food of animals are the carbohydrates, amino acids, proteins, lipids and vitamins. The structure and specific chemical nature of these compounds are controlled by the genes. The genes are responsible for the development of characteristic compounds for different kinds of plants.

Types of Foods of Wild / Zoo Animals

Different kinds of foods required for the feeding of wild/zoo animals can be classified into the following groups:

1. Herbaceous foods: These include tree fodder, shrubs, herbs, forbs, grasses, aquatic plants. Some animal species prefer foliage while some other like flowers, fruits, berries, kernels, seeds and/or tuberous roots. Some wild ruminants also eat succulent bark of trees and tender twigs of shrubs, etc.

   Different lower plants like mosses, lichen, riccia, merchantia, algae (chlorella, spirulina, etc), ferns, palms are eaten by different wild animal species. Yak, reindeer and other herbivorous of snow covered mountains are highly sensitive for smell and dig out forages buried beneath the snow. Yaks obtain feeds by this method during winter migration to relatively warmer climate of lower altitude.

2. Foods of animal sources : Wide range of animals form insects to mammals and eggs to adults are eaten by the carnivorous and omnivorous animals. However, these are not essential in the diets of the omnivorous animals. Some of the common flesh foods of wild animals include most of the herbivorous species, few reptiles, many avian species and fishes found in plenty.

3. Mammalian species as food of wild carnivorous : These include bovines, deer, antelopes, llamoids, caprine, ovine, equine, lagomorphs and rodents, etc. the prey animals for carnivorous predators are variable and depend on their presence in the natural habitats of wild carnivores. Different species of deer and antelopes are common prey. In Africa and Asia, buffaloes are predated. Wild large antelopes, zebra, bison and hippopotamus are common prey of large feline and large reptiles. Sometimes aged elephants and elephant calves are also hunted. Rodent, lagomorphs and other small animals are predated by smaller carnivores and carnivorous avian species such as hawks, owls, eagle and vultures, etc.

Wild carnivorous animals eat total carcass. The large mammals are killed and blood is sucked immediately. The carcass is dragged at hidden place and left for several hours. The carcass is generally eaten at the end of rigor mortis when carcass becomes soft, but hungry animals finish immediately after killing.

Hunting technique is highly variable among the carnivorous animals. Tigers, leopard and cheetah normally hunt alone. Lions, dogs, jackals, wolves and hyena generally hunt in groups. Foxes and many canines prefer left over of other carnivores.

Feeding of Wild animals *in Situ*

The principle of feeding wild animals *in situ* is to provide favourable conditions for the balanced growth of grasslands, herbs, forbs, shrubs and trees. These plants provide fodder for different classes of herbivorous animals. The flowers, fruits, berries, seeds and kernels are mostly used by the omnivorous animals. Herbivorous animals are the common, may be listed as follows:

1. Whole body of mammals : Carnivorous animals prefer the carcass of herbivorous animals. They avoid predation of carnivorous animals.

2. Aquatic animals include fishes, snails, oysters, lobster, crabs and many other species are the foods of carnivores. Kites hunt even the turtles encased in hard shield. The kite lifts a turtle hidden in its shell high in the sky and then drops inverted (hard dorsal side down) on a hard rock. The shell is broken and flesh is exposed for eating.

3. Reptiles, viz. turtles, tortoise, snakes, lizards, etc. are eaten by many carnivorous species.
4. Amphibian species : Frog and its progeny.
5. Worms, viz. cestodes and nematodes from larval to adult stages present in the gut of predated animals.
6. Insects and their larvae include different species of ants, grass hoppers, flies, termites, wasps, their eggs and larvae.
7. Honey is licked by bear of tropical forests.

Foods of carnivorous animals (Fig. 3.1)

Trees and shrubs - Foods of browsing animals

Soil

Grasses, herbs and shrubs - Foods of grazing and browsing animals

Foods of carnivorous animals

Excreta and decaying bones

Soil

Manure

Fig. 3.1 Food cycle of wild animals *in situ*

Factors Requiring Attention of Forest Department Personnel

1. Status of herbage cover, both quantitative and qualitative, of the forest.
2. Pattern of Seasonal Variation in fodder and nutrients supply.
3. Carrying capacity of herbage covers for the herbivorous animals.
4. Carrying capacity of prey (herbivorous animals) for carnivorous animals, natural water sources for drinking, bathing and wallowing and population of carnivorous aquatic animals (if any).

5. Natural water sources for drinking, bathing and wallowing and population of carnivorous aquatic animals (if any).
6. Sources of linking water reservoirs of forest area for drinking water supply during extended droughts threatening minimum water supply for the survival of wild animals.
7. Minerals in the herbages, water and soil and need of supplementation. Deficient minerals are supplied in the form of bricks or blocks. The mineral bricks are placed protected from rains at different places on the grasslands.
8. Injured and weak carnivorous animals : These are dangerous for humans and domestic animals on the periphery of forests. Such animals, particularly the big cats (tigers, leopard, lion, etc) escape to human habitation and hunt humans and domestic animals. Women, children and calves are the easy prey. A man eater is most dangerous because such animals develop liking for such flesh.
9. Hyena and wolves are notorious and they visit villages during dark hours of night. They normally lift goats, kids, sheep and lambs. Human infants and children are also not safe in the periphery villages of forests in habitating wild canines. These are generally nocturnal animals. They come out of burrows in night for lifting small ruminants and human infants. In the forest area they hunt during dawn and dusk when rabbits come out with bunnies for feeding.

Feral dogs, straying in groups in arable fields and on wastelands should not be believed. Incidence of predating children and some times even adult humans is often reported from different states. Such incidences are more common in different parts of India.

Balanced Population Dynamics of Wildlife

Each forest has a carrying capacity for the wild animals, which is affected by the following factors :

1. Herbage cover determines the density of herbivorous animals. Grazing and browsing are balanced by short and long duration periodic movement of the animals. Seasonal migration is quite common in many species of wild animals.

2. Population of common prey like deer, antelopes and lagomorphs determine the number of different predators in the forest.

Any significant increase or decrease in the herbage cover results in corresponding rise and fall in herbivorous and carnivorous animals. Some of the measures required for the balancing among inter-dependent wild lives are :

1. Supply of fodder at different places in the forest.
2. Disposal of surplus herbivorous animals to other forests or markets for human consumption. It is strictly prohibited in India except the periodic elimination of Neelgai from cultivated standing crops. This requires special permission of nominated administrative officer of the district. Probably this provision is not applicable in the Rajasthan state.
3. Translocation of wild carnivorous animals to other forests inhabitating adequate number of prolific prey animals like deer, antelopes, rabbits, and hare, etc.
4. Control of diseases : For this purpose entry of domestic animals is strictly prohibited. Forest workers residing outside are directed to follow hygienic measures strictly. Water of rivers running through the forest is periodically tested for harmful factors.
5. Strict guarding is required for the control of entry of poachers and thieves of fodder and wood.
6. Trespassing of honey collection and medicinal herbage collecting persons should be either prohibited or properly regularized for specific duration.
7. Duties of running forests guards should be rotated frequently.

Selection of foods for Zoo Animals

Different kinds of foods required for the feeding of most of the wild animal species are also eaten by the domestic animals. The foods are procured from the markets. Some problems are faced for the supply of tree fodders with intact branches. This is reasonably compensated by the supply of sugarcane, sorghum, maize and pearl millet fodder. Stovers and kadbies are also fed to many herbivores.

Types of Feeds Required in the Zoo

1. Dry fodder like straws, kadbies, stovers and hay.
2. Green cultivated fodder depending on the cropping season. Common green forages are whole sugarcane, sugarcane tops, green maize, green sorghum, green peal millet, oats, cowpea, berseem and lucerne.
3. Vegetables, roots, tubers and fruits include gourds, leafy vegetables, green chilly, cucumbers, watermelon, muskmelon, carrot, turnips, beets, sweet potato, peaches, lettuce, banana, mango, guava, jack fruits and berries, etc. Raw potato should not be fed and should be boiled or cooked before feeding.
4. Carcass supply : Good quality flesh with bones are supplied for the carnivorous big cats. Chopped flesh is supplied for other carnivores and omnivores.
5. Fresh fishes of different size are supplied for the aquatic reptiles and birds.
6. Compounded feeds of different kinds are supplied for various species of caged animals.
7. Special feeds like jaggrai, honey, balls made of cooked rice, oil, ghee, etc.
8. Minerals and vitamin supplements.
9. Feed additives particularly protective feed additives like probiotics, prebiotics and synbiotics.

Water Requirement

Water is required for drinking, bathing, wallowing, swimming and playing. The common water sources for the wild animals are the rivers, lakes, ponds, canals and streams, etc. The water of natural sources are generally fit for drinking. However, human interference polluted natural water sources to make unfit for drinking. Forest department personnel are required to ensure the control for industrial and sewage pollution of water sources of forests and the rivers flowing through the forest areas.

Zoo animals normally receive water from deep bore wells. Supply of water through the pipelines of town management is also made in some small zoos. However, supply of such water should be avoided due to frequent use of chlorination and other kind of chemical treatments.

The drainage system in the zoo must be maintained in perfect running condition. Water stagnation contaminated with animal excreta provides media for the pathogenic flora (bacteria and fungi) and fauna (enteric protozoa). Some species may use stagnated water in their reach for wallowing and bathing and may expose themselves for external and internal diseases.

Fodder Trees

Several varieties of the tree fodders are available in the rain forests, mangroves sub-temperate leafy trees and conifers, etc. The green leaves, twigs, tender branches, flowers and fruits are included in the diets of wild animals. Most of the wild animals eat leaves, flowers and berries but some wild animal species are very specific, viz. koala feeds on eucalyptus leaves, dromedary camel prefers trees of arid and semi arid zones like babul (*Acacia mylotica*), khejari (*Prosopis sinreria*), neem (*Adzarichta indica*), ber (*Zizyphus jujube*) and many others. Camels in the Indian Thar also eat large quantity of water melon.

Methods of Decontamination of Natural Water Sources in the Wild Animals Habitats

Running water of rivers, streams and water falls are normally suitable for the dinking of the wild animals provided industrial washing and municipal washings are not drained in the direction of flow. If water sources running through the forest are contaminated with organic wastes and heavy metals following measures may be useful in improving the quality of water for the drinking of wild animals:

1. Construction of barriers for reducing the flow rate of running water : This helps silting of suspended organic and inorganic matters. Silting rate depends on the reduction of flow rate and duration before entrance into the forest.
2. Introduction and multiplication of aquatic plants having affinity for the selective absorption of heavy metals, e.g. water hyacinth, duck weeds, hydrilla, pistia and water spinach, etc. wild paddy, reeds and some other species absorb selenium from the water and soil.

3. Culture of small variety of fishes and prevention of capture of frogs, crabs and other aquatic animals helping water purification by eating harmful insects and their larvae.
4. Water of lakes and ponds should be protected from the drainage of industrial and municipal garbage.
5. Different species of algae and other aquatic herbages should be cultured. These plants should be removed periodically from the water sources and disposed at a distant site.
6. Lakes and ponds should also be used for fish culture using mixture of species feeding at different strata from the surface of water to bottom of the water bodies. Other aquatic animals of complementary nature can also be cultured.
7. Periodic removal of silt : Although it is labour intensive but necessary for the maintenance of water quality and water holding capacity of the lakes and ponds. Long delay will limit the water holding capacity and may cause stagnation of rain water in the forest for longer duration due to reduction in water holding capacity of the lakes and ponds. Stagnated water for longer duration may cause pollution due to rottening of fallen leaves and breeding of insect vectors of many infectious diseases.
8. Snails should not be allowed multiplication as many species are intermediate hosts for some stages of life-cycles of fluke worms.
9. Culture of amphibians for the control of insects in and around the water sources.
10. Provide attraction for the aquatic birds. Wild ducks, crane and other large birds eat snails and other crustaseans, which are intermediate host for many helminth parasites and others. Two species of snaila, limnea and endoplanorbis are the intermediate hosts of *Fasciola gigantica* ad *Fasciola hepatica,* etc. these are liver flukes and responsible for wasting disease conditions by damaging hepatic parenchyma and obstructing bile flow by blocking the bile duct.

Common Food Chain of Wild Animals *in situ*

Soil, water, air and solar energy are the sources of nutrients for the growth of plants. Chlorophyll in the green tissues of herbages is evolved for the conservation of solar energy and synthesis of carbohydrates (non-fibrous and fibrous), proteins, lipids and many vitamins or their precursors to be converted into vitamin activity in the animal body. Minerals are absorbed from the soil and present soluble or colloidal in the irrigation water.

The herbages in the forests, ranges and grasslands are eaten by the herbivorous animals. A small quantity of tender leaves, flowers, fruits and seeds are eaten by the simple stomached omnivorous animals. The herbivorous animals are the major foods of carnivorous animals. Omnivorous animals generally feed on dead carcass and left over of large felines.

All animals return considerable nutrients to soil in the form of droppings, urine and decaying carcass. Fallen leaves, damaged plants and decaying trees are also the sources of nutrients for the soil.

Natural Renewal of Herbages

Periodic floods, silting of eroded soil and replacement of soil by storms are the factors responsible for the renewal of soils. Different species of soil micro-organisms draw their nutrients from the decaying organic matter in the soil and convert them into manure suitable for supplying nutrients to the plants. At the same time nitrogen fixing bacteria store atmospheric nitrogen in complex form in the nodules of leguminous and other plant species, which are in turn supplied to the other crops.

Effect of Food Deficit on the Wild Herbivores

Shortage of herbage in the areas of habitat results in change of feeding habits and migration to greener forest or tress passing into the standing cultivated crops. In case of migration territorial conflict occurs among the beasts. The intensity of conflict ranges from mild spar to fierce fight. Elder females play important role in solving the territorial conflict.

In case of feed deficit, wild animals trespass into the standing crops near the forests. Such activities are quite common during the dry season. Although standing crops are grazed and damaged by all wild herbivores but farmers in group manage to minimize the menace of antelopes, cervids and bovines. On the other hand it is very difficult to prevent damage caused by the wild elephants. Hungry and annoyed elephants not only graze the standing crops but sometimes damage the houses and plantation crops. Reports of fatal attack of wild elephants is quite common from the villages near the forest habitated by the elephants in different stages of the India, Nepal, Thailand, Myanmar, Vietnam and Sri Lanka, etc.

Effect of the Food Deficit on Wild Carnivores

During the dry season herbivorous animals move out in search of the feed and water. This causes food deficit for the carnivorous animals. Hungry wild carnivores escape out of the jungle in search of foods. Domestic animals and humans are hunted by these animals. The incidence is quite common in the human habitation near the tropical forests.

Kids, lambs, small domestic animals and human infants are the common and easy prey of small carnivores like jackal, wolves and hyena. Large cats like tiger, leopard and lion hunt domestic cattle, buffaloes and humans. People from farming families particularly ladies, young children and aged people are the easy prey.

Man Eating Behaviour of Wild Carnivores

Tiger, lion and leopard often turn man eater after first hunting. It is said that after eating human flesh these large felines become addict for human flesh. Such felines generally do not return to forest and hide themselves in the vicinity of human habitats around the forests. Sometimes a man-eater feline moves far away from the forest. It has been also seen that some man eaters frequently change their hunting areas. One such recent case of 2014 is that of a tigress from the forests of Himalayan tarai. This tigress created havoc in the areas of Bijnor, Moradabad and Haridwar, etc. Such man eaters re trapped and kept caged in zoo. If it is difficult to catch, such felines are eliminated with the help of hunters.

Wolves, hyena and jackals are known for hunting small animals like sheep, goats, lambs and kids. Pack of feral dogs taking shelter in small forests amidst cultivated fields is very dangerous and has been found to kill and eat not only the animals but also the humans particularly children and ladies. Thus, stray dogs should be pushed into the forests or eliminated from the scene.

Supplements Feeding for Balancing Minerals and Vitamins

Due to great difference in the size and feed intake of herbivorous animals there are scopes of minerals imbalance. Therefore, minerals blocks should be placed at different places in the paddocks for free choice licking. Vitamins are generally mixed in the feeds. Herbivorous animals of tropical countries exposed to sun and fed sun dried or wilted forages normally do not need vitamin supplementation.

Carnivorous and omnivorous animals fed flesh with bones and blood do not need minerals supplementation in normal situation. Weekly feeding of a piece of fresh health liver supply most of the vitamins requirement. However, in the food menu of many zoos vitamin supplements are offered periodically.

Food Management *in Situ*

Animals-plants relationship is responsible for sustaining the wildlife *in situ*. Existence of adequate herbaceous forage, herbivorous animals prey for the carnivorous animals and maximum number of carnivorous and omnivorous animals is necessary for sustaining the balance *in situ*.

The condition *in situ* may be open jungle of tall trees, shrubs, creepers, herbs and grasses or fenced reserves cris-crossed by narrow roads/foot paths for the patrolling on domestic elephants or motor cycles wildlife safari is planned with metalled roads for the driving of closed window vehicles through the animals, particularly the families of big cats. Following steps should be taken for the maintenance of quantitative and qualitative ratio of forages, herbivorous preys and carnivorous and omnivorous animals:

1. In wildlife reserves grassland should be available at different places in the forest. The forest should also have fodder trees and fruit trees alongwith the timber/wood trees. Pasture and fodder trees should be provided in the deep forest and periphery should be avoided specially in areas inhabited by humans and farmers near the boundary of the forests.

Water sources should be also far away from the periphery. Care should be taken to recharge periodically, if the source is not perennial. There should be perfect plan for water supply during prolonged droughts.

Any kind of negligence at the part of forest department management strategies may be the case of food scarcity in the forest for the wild animals. In deficit situation, wild animals move out of the forest area in search of foods. The herbivorous beasts escaping the forest destroy the standing crops. Antelopes and cervids prefer to graze the standing crops, while can of elephants eat and damage orchards of banana and trees of mango, guava, banyan tree, peepal tree, packed tree, gular tree and bael tree, etc.

Escape of herbivorous animals from the forests results in the deficit of prey for the carnivorous animals. This also precipitates in the movement of carnivorous animals out of the forest boundary into the nearby human habitations housing different species of farm animals. Such movement of wild carnivores create dangerous situation for the humans and domestic animals. Small animals like goats, sheep, young calves and human infants and children are lifted away in hides for eating. Large cats like tiger and leopards kill bovines, equines and other animals. Humans, especially ladies and accompanying children on work in the fields are easy prey.

2. In wildlife safari plantation should be designed to provide fodder for herbivorous animals without any considerable break. Patches of grasslands should be available at visible place and short distance from the roads for the tourists vehicles. There should be natural or man made caves at intervals for the shelter of carnivores specially the big cats like lion, tiger, leopard, etc. because these are considered the subjects of more attraction for the tourists safari. The tourists of safari like to see these dangerous wild carnivorous from a short distance.

❑❑❑

4

Feeding Habits of Wild and Zoo Animals

Introduction

Large number of wild animal species have highly varied foods habits due to feed selection, procurement and feeding management of the wild animals in the captive environment of the zoo. The animals are kept for display in the captive conditions of the zoo. These are mostly wild animals but uncommon domestic animals are also translocated from the other areas. The management schedule of zoo animals is prepared on the basis of geo-climatic conditions, food habits and common foods of the local species. These information are the basis of the selection of feeds, preparation of the ration and feeding schedules of different species belonging to mammals, reptiles and avian species evolved for comfortably living in different conditions.

Feeding systems of the animals housed in the zoo is developed on the basis of observations in situ and also the feeds and feeding systems of their domestic cousins and other relatives. This information also helps in finding the alternate foods in the cases of non-availability of the traditional foods.

Types of Animals on the Basis of Food Selection

The organic materials eaten by different species of animals are used for the identification of an animal in the type of food selection. The criteria for classification has been worked out on the basis of the sources of natural edible organic matters constituting more than 60% for the dry matter intake from one or more kinds of the foods. The main constituents of the diets of vertebrates include one or more members of the plants, animals or both. The diets of strict herbivorous or strict carnivorous animals contain more than 90% dry matter of herbages or carcass, respectively.

Followings are the principal classes of animals on the main sources of foods:

a) Herbivorous animals

Large numbers of animal species belong to this group. Different groups of wild and feral animals either consume the whole plant or a specific part of the herbages on their disposal in the forests and wet lands, and on the waste and degraded lands distributed from desert to wetlands and plains of the river basins to hills and mountains of the Bharatiya territory. The herbivorous animals are further sub-grouped into the following two system of food selection and feeding:

1. Classification of the herbivorous animals on the level of feeding on the herbages: The feeding behaviour of the animals depends on the teeth pattern, organ of prehension, mastication system and the segment of microbial digestion in the gastro-intestinal tract. Herbivorous animals collect largest number of bites from different heights of the plants and accordingly they are sub-divided into the following sub-groups:

   i) Ground level feeders : These are grazing animals and occasionally take few bites on the shrubs and trees. These include several species of ovine, bovine, antelopes, equine and cervids.

ii) Middle level feeders : Bovines like mithun (*Bos frontalis*) and gaur (*Bos gaurus*) develop taste for the succulent barks of many shrubs and trees capable of regeneration of the eaten bark. Regenerated bark is more succulent and probably more nutritious due to fresh accumulation of nutrients.

iii) Top level feeders : The herbivorous animals with long neck like camel, cameloids and giraffe are capable to browse on the leaves, flowers and fruits of the shrubs and trees.

The herbivorous animals quickly shift from one level to another level of feeding during non-availability of the feeds of choice.

Another grouping of the herbivorous animals is done on the basis of the part of the herbages preferably eaten by the animals. Preference for a part of plant does not mean that they do not eat other parts of the plants.

2. Classification of the herbivorous animals on the basis of the part of the plant eaten : The herbivorous animals are generally divided into the following groups on the basis of the part of the herbage eaten preferably:

   i) Folivorous animals : The greater proportion of the diets of this group include green leaves. The animals of this group mostly move and feed on the tree leaves. The long neck animals and elephants are folivorous animals.

   ii) Frugivorous animals : The members of this group like to eat the fruits, generally the sweet and succulent berries. Frugivorous animals are mostly primates, frugivorous bats and many species of birds. Ripen neem fruits are also eaten by several species. Ripen fruits of mahua is eaten by humans also.

   iii) Florivorous animals : This group prefers to eat the inflorescence of plants rich in nectar and modified juicy flowers like mahua flower, fig and hypothodium of trees like peepal, gular, pakad and barar.

   iv) Grains, seeds and kernels eating animals : This group is dominated by simple stomach animals of small digestive system of limited food intake capacity. The foods of this group are condensed sources of nutrients. The grains, seeds and kernels are low fibre feeds of generally high feeding value.

The grains and kernels are normally rich in starch, whereas seeds are rich in proteins and oil seeds are rich sources of protein and energy.

b) Carnivorous animals

The animals of this group extract nutrients from different species of invertebrate and vertebrate animals. On the basis of preference, the carnivorous animals are further sub-grouped as follows :

1. Carnivorous animals hunt animals for food. Prey of the carnivorous animals are mostly herbivorous and omnivorous mammals like bovine, caprine, ovine, equine, cervids, swine, lagomorphs and marsupials, etc.
2. Avivorous animals : Some species of carnivorous animals prefer the flesh of many avian species. The ratites and birds in bushes and nests on the trees are the common prey of avivorous animals. Cats, some primates, canines and arborial snakes are avivorous.
3. Ovivorous animals : Many mammals prefer to eat eggs of the avian species and turtles, etc. some aquatic animals eat the spawn of fishes.
4. Piscivorous animals : All animals eating fishes and other aquatic animals are classed as piscivorous animals. Some of animals of this group are dolphins, hippopotamus, whales, crocodiles and several avian species of the wetlands. Piscivorous birds are duck, geese, swan, heron and many others.
5. Insectivorous animals : Different species of insects, their eggs, larvae and pupae are preferably eaten by the animals. Some primates use special technique for eating insects. They put a thin twig inside the insect burrows on termite rocks to collect termites for eating. Most of the avian species eat insects and their eggs, larvae and pupae. Primates can be seen to search and eat lice on the body of other members of group. Herons eat worms, insects and their progeny and for this purpose they can be seen walking behind the ploughing instruments (plough or harrow, etc).

c) Melivorous animals

Some animals like the flavoured sweetness of honey and climb the tall trees for eating honey. Black bear of the tropical forests of

India has been seen to eat honey after blowing away the bees from the honey comb.

d) Nectar eating animal

Some birds with very long, slender and pointed beak suck nectar from the flowers.

Need of Supplements Feeding to Wild Animals

Since wild animals are now national assets and maintained protected under the management of the forest department, it is now responsibility of the forest department to arrange the availability of adequate food and water for the optimum supply of nutrients. The restriction of movements of the wild animals due to gap in the boundaries of different forests, the scope of feed selection from wide range is now limited. The falling of natural trees and replacement of plantation of commercial trees for timber and pulp have limited to scope of selective feeding. Extensive use of monoculture often create nutritional imbalance in the wild animals.

Under changing plantation composition, the responsibility of forest department has increased for the assured supply of foods to wild animals.

Steps Required for the Assured Food Supply and Nutritional Balancing *in Situ*

Following measures should be taken for the assured and uninterrupted supply of wholesome feed and water:

1. Establishment of grassland fields at appropriate intervals in the forest for the grazing of ground level feeders and plantation of edible shrubs and trees for the browsing of middle and top level feeders. Increasing human number, mechanization, deforestation and commercial plantation are some of the factors responsible for ecological disturbances. These changes are disturbing the feed/food sources and nutritional balance. Under such changing conditions there appears to be need of scientific approach for balanced nutritional supply and this can be done by adopting one or more need based methods.

i) Assessment of herbage covers for continuous supply of feeds/ foods. This can be solved by plantation of perennial species and supply of feeds during seasonal scarcity caused by dormant growth of grasses and fall of leaves of deciduous trees and shrubs.

ii) Continuous extraction of soil minerals, deficiency of some minerals occurs in the inmates of the forest. This can be solved by mapping the soil, water and herbage of forest for the status of essential minerals. This problem can be solved by offering multi-minerals lick of required minerals. Starch or molasses or any organic matter containing minerals licks should not be offered during the wet season to avoid the growth of pathogens.

iii) Translocation of surplus animals : On exceeding the carrying capacity of herbages and disturbance between the ratio of predators and preys, the surplus animals are translocated into the other forests of short population.

Processed Feeds for the Captive Animals

For the feeding of herbivorous captive animals in the enclosures of zoo, the compounded feeds for the domestic animals are used for the related animals in zoos. In few cases, minor adjustment is required. Since maintenance of good health is the main objective of the feeding of zoo animals kept in captivity, the medium energy compounded feeds of about 60% total digestible nutrients (TDN) for the adult herbivores and about 65% TDN for the adult omnivorous animals are satisfactory. Crude protein content 9-10% with 60-65% digestibility is adequate for the maintenance of all adult mammalian species.

Breeding is an integrated part of the zoo animals within the limitations of the zoo capacity and scope of translocation within the country and in other countries. Depending on the additional nutritional requirements, the quantity of feed requires 10 to 30% and in case of litter bearing mammals upto 50% increase in the feeding scale.

Specific Essential Nutrient(s) Requirement of Some Wild/ Zoo Animals

Certain species of wild animals need one or more nutrient(s) and sometimes a feed for the maintenance of good health. Prolonged deficiency of certain nutrients may be fatal for the species. Although diets made of several feed ingredients are able to meet the nutritional requirements of most of the species, but some species are known to need specific nutrient(s) for survival. Followings are the known examples :

1. Cobalt is essential for the health and survival of all ruminants because cobalt is essential for the microbial synthesis of cyanocobalamin (vitamin B_{12}).
2. Bulbul and some other citrus fruits eating avian species are unable to synthesize ascorbic acid (Vitamin C) and require dietary supplementation of vitamin C.
3. Dietary supply of taurine is essential for the survival of felines. Before keeping a cat as pet animal, the strict vegetarian families should know that flesh eating is essential for survival.
4. Coprophagy is essential in some species for the supply of amino acids and vitamins. Restriction of coprophage in such species will require regular supply of vitamins and some amino acids.
5. Supplementation of more amount of sulphur is essential in the diets of fibre producing herbivorous animals for the microbial synthesis of sulphur amino acids essential for fibre growth and quality.
6. Fibre (cellulosic feeds and animal fibres) is essential for the normal functions of alimentary tract in the carnivorous animals. Strict carnivores like lion, tiger and others also need fibrous feeds. Many carnivorous animals entire carcass including the body coat and untreated animal fibres are not digested and work as physical factor necessary for stimulating the movement of gut required for propelling the digesta.

Feeding of Herbivorous Mammals

Nature has made enlarged compartments in different zones of the gastro-intestinal (GI) tract. The medium of these enlarged segments is in neutral range for the growth of useful important micro-organisms essential for the synthesis of digestive enzymes for the digestion of cellulosic fibrous feeds. Herbivorous animals do not produce enzymes for the digestion of the cellulosic feeds, the diets of the herbivores.

For the purpose of feeding the life-cycle of the herbivorous animals is divided into three main phases. These phases are (i) milk feeding phase, (ii) transition phase i.e. gradual change of diet from milk to herbaceous feeds and (iii) the phase of herbaceous feeds.

1. Nursing or suckling stage

In mammals the diet starts with the suckling of the mother colostrums, which carries immunoglobulins into the body of the new born infants. This provides protection from many infectious diseases for 3-6 months during which body immune system develops in the growing animals. Whole milk requirement of the infants has been worked out to be about 15% of the body weight for small animals of less than 100kg adult body weight and 10% of body weight for the infants of large body weight during the first month of age. The infants start to eat other feeds and grasses offered to their mothers from second to third week of age. The quantity of milk is reduced to 10 to 7% of body weight during the second month and then gradually stopped in next 7-10 days.

Suckling duration ranges from one month in small animals to more than a year in many large animals. Suckling infants live with the other and nursing duration depends on the lactation length.

2. Transition stage from suckling to common feeds

The suckling infants live with the mother and gradually learn to share the feeds of mother. In situ, the infants follow the dams for grazing and browsing. The intake of herbaceous feeds increases with the corresponding decrease in milk availability.

During this phase concentrate mixture or compounded feed of the dam is gradually increased at the rate of 10% per month upto 50% of the dam's allowance. Forage is also increased at the rate of 5% per month upto 6 months of age.

3. Phase of herbaceous feed

This phase starts after 5 months to 15 months in situ and 5 to 10 months in different species of captive herbivores. The weaned young are separated and fed independently. The rate of feeding includes compounded feed, green forage and dry fodder (hay or straw).

a) Growing animals fed at the rate of 3 kg dry matter per 100 kg body weight. It contains 50% compounded feeds, 25% green forage and 25% dry forage.

b) Finishing period : The amount of compounded feed is either reduced to one third or the total dry matter intake or 1% of dry body weight and remaining 1.5% dry matter is supplied by green and dry fodder.

In natural habitat, herbivorous animals have free choice to select and eat the feeds of choice from the available sources. Free living wild animals extract their nutritional requirements from the natural sources. On occurrence of natural disasters wild animals move to newer pastures. This freedom ends in limits of the zoo enclosures and zoo animals need human intervention for adequate balanced feeding. This is done with the help of feeding standards evolved for the domestic animals of comparable feed choice and digestive system.

Feeding of the Omnivorous Animals

Omnivorous animals are simple stomached animals extracting nutrients from food grains, their milling byproducts, tender leaves, roots, tubers, fruits, kernels and also the foods of animal sources like flesh, fish and eggs, etc. Supplementation of small quantity of foods of animal products are required for the balanced supply of essential amino acids and fat soluble vitamins like A, D, E and K. Processed and sterilized bone meal is good source of minerals. For the purpose of feeding omnivorous mammal can be further divided into the following sub-groups:

1. Swine

The growing phase is divided into three stages of starter, grower and finisher feeds, and the diets of breeding animals. The fibre tolerance of the animals of this group is normally 8-10% but adult can eat feeds of upto 12-13% crude fibre. In wild conditions the animals of this group balance their diets by coprophagy, eating carcass, roots, seeds and tender leaves, etc. in captive conditions of zoo, these animals are fed the standard diets used for different stages of the domestic pigs.

2. Primates

The digestive system of most of the primate species is similar to human but in natural conditions the primates are adopted to eat raw feeds from different sources. These diets include fruits, roots, flowers, seeds, kernels and tender leaves. Many primates eat flesh, eggs, insects, larvae, pupae and fishes, etc.

In the captivity of zoo, the diets of primates normally contain ripen banana, pieces of other fruits, germinated legumes (gram, moong, moth, etc), bread, jaggery, green leaves and fleshy roots, etc.

i) Primate infants share dam's food from 2-3 weeks of age but greater part of nutritional requirements received from suckling the dam.

ii) Growing primates need diets supplying about 18-20% protein and 68-70% TDN on dry matter basis. Milk, milk products and cooked eggs are fed for balancing the requirements of essential amino acids.

iii) Pregnant females are fed 50 to 100% more feed than the diet of adult primates.

The size of different primate species is highly variable and difference in food requirement is large and has been worked out for feeding. The sources of foods differ from one region to another region.

Feeding of the Carnivorous Animals

The greater part of the diet of the carnivorous animals includes flesh. Terrestrial carnivores like, felines and canines are fed the flesh of healthy buffaloes, goats and sheep. Small quantity of green leaves, fruits and bread, etc. are eaten by some species. Since flesh is offered with intact bones, minerals supplementation is normally not required. Vitamins are supplied periodically. Feeding of fresh liver and other glandular tissues meets the requirements of almost all vitamins.

Aquatic animals and the animals of wet lands prefer fishes, crabs, lobsters and molasses. These are very good sources of major and minor nutrients. For the supply of carbohydrates, these animals consume some amount of aquatic plants. In addition to carbohydrates, aquatic herbages also supply proteins, vitamins and minerals.

Feeding of the Geriatric Animals

Geriatric wild animals are rarely seen in the forest because increasing age reduces the physical strength due to which such animals become easy prey of the carnivorous animals. However, in captivity of zoo, these animals need easily digestible foods. In some cases, geriatric animals may need cooked foods and higher dose of vitamins.

Very old animals with shed teeth are fed semi-solid and liquid feeds in the form of slurry, soup and licks, etc. Juicy fruits, ripen banana and many other soft and succulent forages are fed to herbivores and omnivores.

Feeds and Feeding of Sick Animals

Palatable, easily digestible and nutritious foods are used for the feeding of sick animals. The physical form of the feeds depends on the kind of sickness:

1. In case of fever, palatable liquid feeds are offered after cooling.
2. In case of oral inflammation non irritant and nutritious liquid feed is offered.
3. In case of gastro-enteritis/enteritis the feeds should be palatable, succulent and easily digestible.
4. Parental feeding is required for the patients unable to swallow the feeds.
5. Rectal feeding is used for the feeding of large quantity of liquid feeds.

❑❑❑

5

Balanced Soil-water-air-solar Energy-plant-animal Relationship for Sustaining Wild Animals *in Situ*

Introduction

Soil is a dynamic complex compound and basic source of nutrients for all the living creatures on the earth. The living creatures may be plant or animals ranging from invisible microscopic flora and fauna to tall trees and mammoth elephants. Soil has little nutritional value for the herbage in absence of water and air which is the major source of carbon, nitrogen and oxygen. The three basic factors of nutrients and nutrients utilization by the plants and animals are inseparable for the existence of the herbages. The herbages are major foods of the animals. The plants and their products (grains, fruits, flowers) and animals and their products (flesh, milk, eggs, honey, etc) are the foods of animals. Excreta voided by the animals and decaying herbages are again added into the soil, which enrich soil with organic and inorganic nutrients.

Soil

It is the basic requirement for the existence of life on the earth. The dependence of life on the earth may be direct and indirect. Majority of herbages receive larger amount of nutrients from the soil. The soil is a complex mixture of elements, organic and inorganic compounds and microorganisms. Soil microorganisms play significant role in the nutritional enrichment of soil by decaying the fallen leaves, plants and animals. The microbial action converts fallen organic matter into the humus, which is an important source of carbon, nitrogen and minerals for the growth of the herbages.

Water

Water is an important solvent for dissolving the soluble nutrients and an essential medium for the utilization of nutrients for the synthesis of organic compounds required for the formation of tissues. The common compounds synthesized for the growth of plants are the amino acids and proteins, fatty acids and fats, carbohydrates consisting of sugars, starch and fibrous complex carbohydrates and lignin. The other constituents are pigments, vitamins and minerals. The basic chemicals of the life are transported into the plant by roots through the process of ascent of sap and imbibitions of the aqueous solution of the nutrients contained in the soil.

Air

Carbon dioxide, oxygen and nitrogen are the main constituents of air utilized by the plants. Normally green plants inspire carbon dioxide and expire oxygen during the night. Carbon, oxygen and hydrogen are the constituents of carbohydrates (carbon and hydros). These are also the constituents of the simple fats. In addition to carbon and water, protein synthesis also requires nitrogen. Another important role of air is the dispersal of seeds. Light weight and wing seeds of grasses, shrubs and trees are carried by air from one place to another place. The distance covered depends on the speed and direction of air movement.

Sunlight or Solar Energy

Solar energy is responsible for the occurrence of biochemical reactions in the plants. Chlorophylls and some other pigments of the live plants are responsible for the utilization of solar energy for storage in the organic forms like carbohydrates, lipids, proteins and vitamins.

Plants

Herbages growing on the soil are the foods of animals. Herbivorous and most of the omnivorous animals extract their nutritional requirements from the herbages. While feeding on the natural herbages animals disperse nutrients for the plants in the form of urine, faeces and saliva. The animals also help in the dispersal of seeds attached on their bodies or hard kernels retaining germination potential even after the actions of the digestive juices.

Territorial Behaviour of the Wild Animals

The forest type, herbage cover, water resources, seasonal variation and human interference are some of the important factors affecting the territorial behaviour of the animals. Co-existence of flora and fauna determines their existence. Under normal conditions wild animals live within the limits of their habitat. The groups or families of different species are controlled and lead by a leader or a group of leaders in different hierarchy. Each species mark their territory and there is little trespass in normal conditions of food supply. Groups and families of herbivorous, carnivorous and omnivorous animals live together in separate areas with mutual understanding.

Different parts of the day has been adapted by different species for feeding and movement. The period of activities may be dawn, forenoon, afternoon, dusk or night. These periods have been adapted on the basis of long experience of numerous generations for protection from the enemy (predators). Inspite of danger of predation the three broad groups of herbivorous, carnivorous and omnivorous animals live together on a common natural herbage cover ranging from grassland to wetland, forests, hills, mountains and sea coasts, etc. This system is continuing due to natural balance. The herbivorous animals normally follow periodic rotation in their territory. The predators normally catch one or two animals at a time as per their requirement. A running group of deer chased by a large cats (Tiger, Lion, Cheetah, etc.) halts spontaneously after the predation of a member. Dudhwa national park in the Himalayan Tarai in Bharat (India) is a rain forest of tall growing sal, sagaun (teak) and other species. It has large and small patches of grasses, different kinds of bushes, wetlands, lake and a river flowing through the park. In the park common herbivores are swamp deer, spotted deer, hog deer, black buck and Neelgai. Dominant species are spotted deer and swamp deer. Tiger and leopards are the main predators. Spotted deer and swamp deer herd during night on the high ground away from the dense forest. Grazing hours start at dawn and animals move to water sources around mid day. Birds and monkeys raise alarm for the presence of a predator (tiger/leopard). The leading stage thumps its forelegs on a hard group and signals the group for safe running. The running group is chased by the tigers for some distance. Once a member is caught, they stop, look helpless for few minutes and then move slowly and free from tension but alert.

Trespassing on Neighbouring Standing Crops

Due to fall in grass cover during the dry season, the herbivores frequently trespass for feeding on the standing crops. This is an annual seasonal problem of the farmers of the boundary of forests inhabited by the wild herbivorous animals. The movement of wild herbivores on the standing cultivated crops creates two main problems for the local people : (i) The crop is not only grazed but also laid on the ground due to movement and playing and (ii) These animals are followed by the predators and humans become the easy prey. The large cats (tiger and leopard) kill adult men and women, and the wild canids (wolves and jackals), lift infants, children and small animals (goats, sheep and young calves).

Seasonal Migration

Seasonal migration of wild animals is a routine practice in some areas. The causes of seasonal migration are (i) the drastic fall in the carrying capacity of the herbage cover and (ii) non-availability of drinking water due to drying of the seasonal water sources. In the Kewaladeva Bird Sanctuary water supply during dry season is maintained by draining canal water in the lake of the park. Few tube wells are also operated in different parts of the park. Long distance international and national seasonal migration is more common among the birds. Seasonal movement of elephant herds in the south and south-east Asia is quite common. The Asian elephants move in the forests of Bharat (India), Nepal, Bhutan, Bangladesh and Myanmar. The another territory of elephants movements extends in south part of Odisha, Jharkhand, Chhattisgarh, east part of Maharashtra, Madhya Pradesh and Andhra Pradesh. The elephant herds of south India normally move in the forests of south part of Andhra Pradesh and Maharashtra, and the forests of Karnataka, Kerala and Tamil Nadu.

Natural Factors Affecting Wild Animals Population

Food, water and shelter are the basic requirement for the survival of the wild animal species of the highly diverse food habits. Good soil moistened by the adequate rain fall and solar radiation energy support lush growth of herbages necessary for the existence of animals. Followings are the major natural factors affecting the types and population of the wild animals. The large savannah grassland of Africa crossed by Congo river is the homeland of the wild African buffaloes. Some of the important dynamics of wild animals can be listed as follows:

Requirements of the herbivorous animals

Common herbivorous wild animals of Bharat are antelopes like black buck, chinkara and neelgai, deep species like spotted deer, swamp deer, hog deer, barking deer and sambhar, etc., large herbivores like elephants, rhinoceros, wild buffaloes and gaur, and small like hare and rabbits. The other wild herbivorous species found in small number and endangered include Thar of Neelgiri, long horn sheep and goats of Himalaya of Jammu and Kashmir province, cheru of Sikkim area and wild ass of Kutchh region. These are almost strict herbivorous animals which start feeding by suckling the dam's mammal. The suckling starts within short time of birth and after some time of springs are gradually weaned to herbages.

The species of herbivores and their density on the grasslands and forests depends on the type of vegetation. The population and rate o multiplication of herbivores affect the species and number of the carnivorous animals. The factors affecting animal composition in wild can be summarized as follows :

1. Herbage cover : Forests of dense population of all trees, embracing luxuriant climbers, scattered bushes and patches of different kinds of grasses provide foods for different species of the herbivorous animals ranging from tiny rodents, rabbits and hare to heavy elephants and rhinoceros.

2. Perennial water sources : Water is an important factor affecting the existence of wild animals. The composition of wild animals is significantly affected by the type of water sources. Elephant, swamp deer (Barasingha), rhinoceros and wild buffaloes are found in the vicinity of perennial rivers, large natural lakes and perennial wetlands for bathing and wallowing.

   Deep perennial water is the habitat of aquatic animals like crocodile, turtles, tortoise, dolphins and many others. Most of the aquatic species thrive on each other but few also hunt strangers visiting the water bodies. Stories of predation of cattle, other animals or even humans by crocodiles is quite common.

3. Shelter : Different kinds of shelters are used by different species. Most of the deer species like cheetal, sambhar and barasingha retire on open upland. Antelopes like black buck, chinkar and neelgai prefer plains and feed on cultivated crops. Some times neelgai population becomes pest in most parts of Uttar Pradesh, Tarai of Uttrakhand, Haryana, Punjab, some parts of Madhya Pradesh and other provinces.

Monkeys, squirrel and most of the avian species rest on trees and holes in trees. Birds fabricate nests of different characteristic designs from dry grasses. One such example is the nest of Baya bird hanging from the tree branches on the grasslands of tropical region. Dense bushes are the shelter for hog deer and hare, etc. and many avian species.

Rabbits, canines and rodents live underground in the burrows of their characteristic layouts, burrows are generally made on uplands in the areas of trees. Some wild animals like jackal, hare and porcupine also live in the non-forest areas.

4. Scope of migration during adverse situation : Seasonal changes in herbage cover and destruction of food resources during disaster require migration to comfortable areas for food and water. Most species possess natural sense. The most common example is the migration of birds in winter season from temperate zone to tropical zone. Movement of elephant families from one forest to another forest or frequently on cultivated crops.

5. Cultivation of preferred crops : Many wild animals particularly monkeys and frugivorous avian species move in orchards and feed on fruits. Fresh fruit eating containing high amount of vitamin C is essential for the survival of bulbul because they are unable to synthesize vitamin C (ascorbic cid). Elephants like sugarcane, banana and lush growing food grain crops. Jackals feed on sugarcane and maize ears at milk to dough stage. Porcupines like potatoes and sweet potato.

6. Presence of human predators : Most of the wild animal species are capable of understanding the mind set of humans. Frequent visits of hunters with fire arms and other hunting weapons and use of these appliances for hunting have developed a sense of fear from the humans. It is frequently referred that African wild buffaloes hate humans. They are revengeful and charge to fatal end. The black large species of African wild buffalo, Syncerus caffer is called "Black death" and annual casualities before restriction of humans in Savannah were 300-400.

Large cats (tigers, lion, leopard, etc) and crocodiles hunt humans in their approach. It is said that once a large cat cats human flesh, it develops preference and becomes man eater. Farmers, herdsman and strangers in the Himalayan tarai of Uttrakhand and Uttar Pradesh are occasionally predated. Small children and infants are predated by the wolves, jackals and feral dogs. Sometimes society cats and mongoose also skill infants.

Role of Air, Water and Animals in the Growth of Herbage

The dispersal of seed, seedlings and even the intact plants is carried by the air movement. Wing seeds and light weight tiny seeds are dispersed by the air from one place to another place. Heavier seeds are carried by high speed air. The seeds, thus dispersed, germinate and proliferate at the new place, if agro-climate is favourable.

Floating seeds and fruits are carried by the flowing water from one place to another. The seeds lodged on the banks enroute establish at the new place in favourable conditions.

Animals particularly birds carry seeds in alimentary tract and attached on the body for long distance. Seeds of many plants specially the tiny seeds of *Ficus spp.* and stone seeds of guava, etc. retain their germination potential even after retention in the gastrointestinal tract for 6 hours to 40 hours. During passage cross the gastrointestinal tract these seeds also pass through the different biochemical reaction media of gastric juice, intestinal secretions, pancreatic juice and bile providing media of about pH 2 to 7 or so. The dispersal of seeds helps in the exchange of new plant species.

Natural Activities for Balancing Ecology

Ecological balancing is essential for the existence of all kinds of living creatures on the earth in mutual co-existence. Nature uses its resources in a manner to provide congenial environment on the earth and its environment. Water, air and temperature together prepare soil for the proliferation of micro-organisms to make the soil suitable for the growth of numerous species of plants on the earth. Significant parts of these plants provide food for most species of animals. Considerable portion of plants again returns to soil to be again mixed with the soil. Animals are also the foods of animal. The complete cycle of different kinds of microbial, plant and animal lives may be considered a complex form of mutual parasitism. It is considered that the life of parasites normally depends on the life of the host. Therefore, parasites do not like to kill the host. Same principle is applicable for the existence of all kinds of life on the earth.

Natural factors play important roles for the balancing of ecology. Heavy rains, periodic droughts, storms, avalanche, hail storm and lightening, etc. change the environment from time to time. However, industrial revolution from the eighteenth century has disturbed the global environment tremendously during the twentieth century due to fast pollution of environment. This has significant adverse effects on the living creatures on the earth.

Recycling of Nutrients in the Wild

The plants and animals in the jungle born and vanish in the native soil. Little volatile substances are taken away or added by the air movement as air has no boundary. Addition of matter particularly the inorganic salts are generally nominal in the native soil but significant in the industrial areas and brick cleans producing large amount of fumes impregnated with carbon and inorganic matters. The contamination of the forest soil depends on the kind of emittance of polluted fumes and pollutants in the fumes.

In non-contaminated jungle little changes occur in the soil and biological composition. The herbages are eaten by the herbivores and undigested portion is returned to soil. The herbivores are eaten by the carnivores and undigested portion is returned to soil. The gases emitted by the animals are mostly used by the herbages.

Control of Water Pollution

The water bodies of the forest should be kept free from man-made pollution. Industrial effluents, municipal garbage and any other organic or inorganic wastes should not be drained into water bodies running across the forests reserves of wild animals.

Utilization of Services of Vanvashi for Wild Animal Protection and Conservation

The families living in the vicinity of wildlife reserves should be educated to be part of the wild animals protection and conservation team. These families may help actively from the chronic menace of poachers against a limited facility of fuel wood for cooking, forage for few livestock and some wood or bamboo for replacement of huts. The families should be registered with the forest office and the movement of any member away from the home should be informed in the forest office. Arrival of new relatives and strangers should be informed in the forest office. They should be allowed honey collection on feasible booster basis, viz. 50% share or so.

Role of Humans in Environmental Disturbances

Human being has made wonderful discoveries for their welfare. For a longtime it could not be visualized by the researchers that all comfort providing inventions are also responsible for the environmental pollution. These changes have evolved many harmful factors specially the newer pathological micro-organisms and harmful chemicals. These harmful complexes are a threat for all kinds of the life on the earth.

Now it is high time for the humans to rationalize their activities for the protection and conservation of different kinds of lives on the earth. Some of the most important factors responsible for creating imbalance and disturbances on the earth may be listed as follows:

1. Indiscriminate deforestation.
2. A forestation without considering the social, economical and ecological consideration.
3. Forest development with least consideration of grasslands, shrubs and fodder tree for the herbivorous animals, fruits for the primates and many avian species and perennial water bodies for the aquatic animals.
4. Improper and limited control on poaching.
5. Probably there is no provision of exchange or translocation of eligible males of threatened species from one forest to another forest.
6. Increasing encroachment of forest lands for farming and other purposes.
7. Construction of offices and guest houses for tourist within the wildlife centres, parks and reserves. Guest houses are often constructed at different places inside the deep forest.
8. Frequent movement of oil energy using vehicles for the tourists. It is a major source of air, water and herbage pollution.
9. Lack of proper education on the management of the wild animals in situ, in zoological gardens and under limited area in wildlife.
10. Extensive use of aluminum foil and polyethylene bags for carrying edible products in the forests and zoological gardens.
11. Inspite of strict instructions for not offering any kind of foods, people do not hesitate to do so. On pointing out by the zoo officials and forest guards, they simply utter sorry.
12. Tourists visiting wildlife sanctuaries and National Wildlife parks frequently carry soft drinks, fruit juice and beverages made up

of milk. After using the empty containers are often disposed of carelessly. Even few residual drops of beverages in these containers are good media for the multiplication of pathogenic micro-organisms. Sometimes, a pathogen becomes highly dangerous and may be epidemic.

Preventive Measures for Minimizing Health Hazards Caused by Foods in the Zoo

Following steps should be strictly taken for the prevention of health hazards to zoo inmates:

1. A zoo should have two step entrances with a gap of about 5-6 meters width between the outer and the inner gate.
2. There should be a shallow walking passage between the two gates. The shallow ally must contain a suitable antiseptic of optimum strength.
3. No food and water should be allowed inside the zoo. However, milk and medicated water for the infants and geriatrics can be allowed with the condition of not disposing of any container and left over of foods and beverages.
4. There should be controlled hygienic canteens in proper enclosures and preventive measures for the access of rodents, birds and cats, and also for the insects, cockroach and beetles, etc. to possible extent.

Human Hazard of Nutritional Importance for the Zoo/Captive Animals

Inspite of instructions at the entrance of zoo and at prominent places in the zoo, many visitors fail to restrain themselves and bring edible inside the zoo. People visiting the zoo often offer foods to primates, lagomorphs, rodents and birds. Some people also offer breads to deer, antelopes and other animals. This is an unwanted habit of humans and many times such foods become hazardous for the zoo animals. In tropical summer green cucumber and spoiled melons may cause infection.

People visiting from the rural areas of animal rearing groups may also transmit infection, particularly that of the zoonotic diseases. In no case, left over foods contaminated with saliva should be offered to zoo inmates. The empty packets, ice cream cups and other disposables should always be disposed off in the dustbins kept at different places in the zoo.

Canteen Inside the Zoo

There should not be any canteen inside the zoo because it is difficult to control the access of rodents, squirrel, cockroach, ants, etc. these are potential hazards responsible for the contamination of the food items.

Only wholesome drinking water should be available inside the zoo. There should be strict instructions to mothers for the judicious and safe use of milk for their infants. Milk should not be disposed of in the dustbins, feeding bottles should not be washed inside the zoo and disposable milk polypacks should be disposed off only in the dustbins placed outside the habitats of the zoo animals.

Inspite of such limitations it is not practical to restrict food, water and medicine intake on humanitarian grounds. Therefore, department should provide restaurant facilities through standard contractors under the strict supervision of the forest personnel including the forest veterinarian and sanitary staff.

❑❑❑

6

Behaviour of Wild Animals Affecting Feeding in Captivity and *in Situ*

Introduction

In the wild environment of the forests, hills, mountains, deserts and water bodies different classes of terrestrial, amphibian and aquatic animals of highly diversified nature live together in great mutual relationship. In wild herbivorous animals are fully aware that life is uncertain and they have to live in the ecological conditions of the habitat. It is evident from the habitation of herbivorous, omnivorous and carnivorous in the same forest. In aquatic bodies all plants, omnivorous aquatic animals and carnivorous aquatic animals live together. There is another situation of terrestrial and aquatic animals' co-existence. Terrestrial animals in such situation are fully aware with the danger of predation by the aquatic carnivores like crocodiles, and alligators, etc., but they frequently visit water bodies for drinking, bathing, wallowing and sometimes feeding on the aquatic herbages. During this period, one, two or more animals are frequently predated by the aquatic carnivores.

Wild-wild predation can be seen in the television programmes on the wild animals of different ecological composition of various countries spread between the poles on either side of the equator.

Feeding Behaviour of Mammalian Infants

There are no defined teats in the primitive mammals and milk is secreted through scattered glands on the abdominal surface on either side of the mid line. In the marsupials like kangaroo the milk gland is situated inside the abdominal pouch. The gestation period in kangaroo is only about 30 days and foetal delivered is still in the embryonic stage. Probably characteristic phenomenon guides the embryo to travel into the abdominal pouch, where it attaches with the teat until complete development.

In the higher mammalian species gestation period ranges from 30 days to more than 1 year in many large species. The animals of this group possess well organized mammary glands for drainage of milk through the teats. The mammary glands develop into the females during the puberty. The secretary parenchyma of the mammary glands grows very fast during the terminal stage of pregnancy. In normal animals, milk secretion starts alongwith parturition to provide colostrums (first milk) to new born within few minutes.

Types of Well Developed Mammary Glands

The mammalian species of this large group can be classified on the basis of the habitat and the location of the mammary glands on the body.

1. Classification of mammals on the basis of habitats

These animals can be classified into the following three groups:

a) Arborial : These mammals mostly live at a place of the ground surface. The habitat is normally marked. Cavities of different shape and size on these, cavities and caves on the hills and the forsa on the ceilings, domes and other places of abandoned buildings are used for housing by different species. Most of the classes of this group prefer a dark place. Some of the species are bats, monkeys and squirrel, etc.

b) Terrestrial : Largest groups are terrestrial and live in the bushes, caves, plains, woodlands, hills, mountains and arid lands.

c) Mammalian of wetlands : Many mammals have developed amphibian behaviour living in water and swamp or on the ground for almost equal time. These are wild buffaloes, swamp deer, otter and rhinoceros, etc.

d) Aquatic mammals : These species always live in water and they can not survive for longer period in non-aquatic habitat. Among these also few live in fresh water and some other live in saline water. Some examples are the dolphins and whales.

2. Classification of the mammals on the basis of location of mammary glands on the ventral aspect of the body

The mammary glands are always found in pairs. Any deviation is the natural freak born rarely due to genetic abrasion or any other factor. The location of mammary glands depends on the species and these are three distinct regions:

a) Thoracic or pectoral mammary glands : These are invariably a single pair normally located on either side of the midrib and almost between the fore limbs. A large number of wild animals belong to this group, viz. all primates, elephants.

b) Abdominal (thoraco-abdominal) mammary glands : These are present from thoracic region to inguinal region in pairs ranging from 4 to 6 pairs in most of the species. The examples are canine, feline, swine, rodents and lagomorphs. The number of teats is considered the maximum natural litter size of species. Normally litter size is smaller than the maximum capacity. In rare cases litter size is larger than the maximum capacity, i.e. the total number of the teats. The udder size suddenly enlarge during the terminal phase of pregnancy and before parturition (farrowing, whelping or kindling) the teats are enlarged, engorged, bright pink and prominent. After delivery each infant hold a teat and teats suckled by the offsprings remain functional and appears prominent. The remaining non-suckled teats regress in few days. In some animals one or more active and aggressive infant suckle more than one teat. In such cases the number of functional teat is more than the litter size.

c) Inguinal mammary glands : This develops as a single organ containing 2 or 4 glands in equal number from either side of the mid line. These are further divided into two sub-groups:

   i) Mammary glands of two halves, each draining through independent well developed teat. Examples are antelopes, cervids, caprine, ovine and equine.

   ii) Mammary glands of four independent quarters separated by inter glandular septa. Each gland drains through long teat. Common examples are bovine, camelids and llanmaids.

Nursing Behaviour of Wild Mammals

The system of breast feeding is highly variable among the wild animals. The difference is significant among the herbivorous, omnivorous and carnivorous species, and also between the single young and litter producing mammals. Litter size also affects the nursing behaviour of the mammals.

1. Nursing behaviour of herbivorous mammals

Almost all species of the herbivorous mammals feed their off springs in standing position. Mothers also guide their infants for changing the teats for suckling. The dams normally call their infants on increasing the pressure of udder due to fast multiplication of lactocytes and different quantity of milk (cisternal milk) in various species being a little in wild Asian buffaloes (*Bubalus bubalis*) and quite large quantity in wild cattle (*Bos indicus*) and gaur (*Bos gaurus*), etc. Some native tribal people sometimes claim the collection of coagulated milk from the forests. In most, whereas, says such products are considered the coagulated milk of gaur.

On engorgement of the teats and udder, goats stop browsing and grazing and give a call to kids or walks to kids. A goat nunny with triplets and larger litter size (rare in wild goats) manage proportionate nursing to all kinds.

Buffalo calves also suckle from the posterior aspects through the space between the hindlimbs during grazing on the ranges.

The fawns of antelopes and deer species nurse in standing position. Twinning is quite high in neelgai.

She camel is not disturbed by suckling and continues browsing on tall trees and shrubs.

Once the udder is suckled, the dams move forward. Sometimes they push away the infants, some use milk lick and sometimes scold affectionately like a mother.

From television channels the affectionate and protective behaviour of lactating wild elephants. The pair of breast is pectoral and calf suckles from the side.

Nursing duration ranges from 4-6 months in the caprine and ovine to 6-12 months in bovines and more than a year in the camels, African buffaloes, elephants and rhinoceros. With the increase in age, dams guide grazing and browsing. Mouth to mouth contact during the grooming the calf by licking, grazing and browsing introduce the taste of herbages in the off springs. This is the source of rumen contamination by the natural symbiotic micro-organisms of the ruminants and the non-ruminant herbivorous animals.

In the initial stage ruminal micro-organisms acclimatize in the internal environment of the developing rumino-reticulum type compound stomach systems. These ruminal microorganisms gradually increase activities with the simultaneous increase in the herbage intake. High intake of milk delays the development of microbial digestion. In natural habitat development of the rumen digestion and metabolism takes 3 to 6 months in different species being shorter in small species and longer in large species. Low milk production also favours early ruminal development due to increased intake of herbaceous feeds.

2. Nursing behaviour of the litter producing herbivorous lagomorphs

Lagomorphs deliver litter of 6-12 bunnies, which are blind in early life in rabbit. Pheromone is considered to guide the bunnies to engorged teats. The doe also guides her bunnies for suckling. The process occurs in lying position. At the time of feeding them gives call to the infants and lies on the side exposing the udder and teat. During the suckling period bunnies are also guided by the legs and the dam attempts to provide equal opportunity each baby.

3. Nursing behaviour of the litter producing omnivores

Wild pigs deliver litters of 4 to 16 piglets in different species. In the normal course suckling occurs in lateral recumbancy but grown up piglets can be seen dragging by the moving dam while suckling. Swine females normally do not nurse in standing position.

4. Nursing behaviour of the carnivorous mammals (canines and felines)

Wild canines and felines deliver litter of blind pups and cubs, respectively. Opening of the eyes of infants takes 14-21 days. The lactating mother gives call to babies and allow suckling in lateral recombant posture. Aggressive babies attempt to push away the weaklings for suckling more teats. However, dams attempt to correct the behaviour of aggressive babies and encourage and guide the weaklings by her legs. Sometimes the dam rebukes and pushes away the dominant off springs. During the terminal phase of the nursing period the dams may allow suckling in standing position.

5. Nursing behaviours of the primate

Normally single baby is delivered by a primate. The baby becomes active immediately after the colostrums feeding. Nursing is done by the mother in sitting posture. She holds young baby in arms during the nursing period. The baby is guided to suckle both teats alternatively during the suckling duration. The baby is also groomed and cleaned at the time of suckling. The dam also attempts to remove the ectoparasites, if any, and licks bruises, etc. for healing. During movements, baby is carried on the back. Sometimes very young baby can be seen suckling during the movement. The baby holds the dam with the help of arm's and legs, callipered around the body of the mother.

6. Feeding behaviour of dam dependent chicks

The chicks of large number of the avian species are incompletely formed at the time of hatching. The chicks of such species are unable to identify, pick and engulf foods as seen in the chicks of sparrow, parrot and many other avian species. These chicks are mouth to mouth fed by the mother, father or both in different species.

In case of ratites specially the rhea, the father takes the responsibility of incubation, feeding and rearing in early life. The female mates with several males during the breeding season and she does not bother for the babies. Sometimes she runs in search of another male while still laying the previous clutch. Such stray eggs are called orphan eggs and may be fertile also.

Natural Relationship for Safety and Feeding Amongst Wild Species

The life of wild animals is a system of co-existence of preys and predators in the same forest. The predators are carnivorous and sometimes omnivorous animals, and the preys are mostly herbivorous and rarely omnivorous animals. The interdependence of herbage, herbivores and carnivores in a balanced system is responsible for sustaining ecology of the forests.

There is well designed communication system amongst the arborial and terrestrial animals of the forests. Avian species, monkeys and other nimals moving from ground to trees and flying in the sky always keep an eye on the movement of different species in the forest. Sight of a big cat (lion, tiger and leopard) is quickly communicated by emitting characteristic alarming vocalization. The leaders of the herds and flocks of herbivorous (common prey) animals become alert and give directions for safe movement and hiding. The large cats normally kill only one animal at a time for food. Once an animal is killed the running and straying animals (prey) stop for a while to mourn the death of fellow habitant. After this routine activities start as usual.

Another example of coordination is observed in feeding behaviour. During fodder scarcity in dry season monkeys pluck and throw leaves and fruits for the herbivores clustering beneath the trees.

Sense Organs and Food Search

Sense of smell and sight helps the search of foods. Herbivorous animals search the forages of preference by smell. During movement amidst forest the frequently grazed grasses and browsed trees can be identified by new sprout. Non-grazed and less grazed forages are found covered with mature leaves and only few scattered new leaves. However, this appearance is not applicable to deciduous trees and other plants.

Wild animals are also capable to search the newer sources of water before the complete drying of the available sources. International and inter-continental movement and migration of the animals is well established for the search of foods and water. Wild elephants and other animals frequently move from one country to another across the jungles and grassland of south and south-east Asian countries. Large number of Siberian birds in winter fly to warmer zones of the earth. These birds often fly out of the Asian countries to different parts of Australia, Africa, South America and many islands of warmer zones. Serial studies have shown that most of the birds prefer to visit the same site every year.

There are also evidences of hereditary traits for the preference of the habitat. For example, the green turtles travel from coastal area of Tamil Nadu to seashore of Odisha for egg laying the females cover their eggs beneath the sand for hatching and then return back to south. The newly hatched young turtles automatically move to join the group in south without the help of any guide. Likewise, Hilsa fish moves to sea from spawning and the fry return back to sweet water of rivers for growing and living.

Seasonal movement of feed and water is an annual feature. These beast are aware with the place and migration is guided by the experienced leaders. However, during extended long duration, severe droughts heavy mortality due to starvation is not uncommon. Such mortality further creates health hazards due to proliferation of the pathogenic micro-organisms.

Inherent Traits in Wild Animals for Balancing the Diets

Deficiency of nutrients below the critical level increases craving for the deficient nutrients. This results in depraved appetite. Such incidence is more prevalent during the scarcity caused by natural disasters causing destruction of feed and water sources. Even in apparently adequate forage supply in many forests mineral deficient feeds result in the intake of mineral rich clay and bones, etc. Mud/clay holes are common in the minerals deficient forests. Large herbivorous beasts of minerals deficient forests consume mineral rich clay, rock and saline/alkaline soils.

Development of Deprived Appetite for Survival

Deficiency of minerals and other nutrients is the cause of deprived appetite. This results in the abnormal feeding like coprophagy, urine dinking, chewing of decaying bones and delaying woods. This change frequently becomes the cause of infectious diseases. Deficit of forages causing acute hunger often results in the intake of hazardous herbages that grow lush in drought hit areas.

Occurrence of Cannibalism

Deficiency of nutrients, particularly minerals and vitamins, results in cannibalism. The disorder is more common in the carnivorous and omnivorous animals. Some times it is observed in the domesticated animals like sows, bitches and queens reared in the confinement of intensive management. Occurrence of cannibalism is not expected in wild animals because they try to balance the deficiencies by eating uncommon matters from different natural sources in the forest. Incidence of cannibalism is sometimes observed in the females kept in the confined housing of zoos.

The causes of cannibalism may be supply of faulty feeds, imbalanced feeds or abnormally size litter. All these factors are the causes of deficiency and acute deficiency of certain nutrients is the cause of deprived appetite. Such clinico-pathological changes are more common in the large litter bearing females. Litters of such females contain more than normal number of infants, weaklings, immature infants or still birth. The rate of foetophagy is generally very rapid and in no time dam eats her total litter and placenta.

Feeding During Captivity

After capture and housing in the enclosure of zoos the wild animals are deprived of the freedom of feed selection of feeds. The captive animals depend on the calculated diets of few feeds large available in the market for procuring. Inspite of certain limitations efforts are made to provide the feeds of choice to the possible extent but in most of the zoos, it is difficult to provide large space and more number of animals of more than one species considered to produce competition for feeding. Such competition amongst the species increases appetite and voluntary feed intake.

Recently captured wild animals housed individually in a limited area of enclosure time for adjustment. The change in normal behaviour is visible. Most of the new captures becomes aggressive, restless and off feed. The frequency of urination and defecation increases but quantity decreases. Feeding and dinking are resumed on the onset of hunger and thirst, and it takes several days to resume optimum intake of feed and water. Once the new inmate is adapted in the new environment of its enclosure, it should be fed as per the requirement. Adaptation becomes easier on housing the new entrant close to older inmates of same or related species.

Captive animals of zoo are fed as per the ration schedule suggested by the animal nutritionists in the zoo. Following factors should be kept in mind for optimum feeding of the zoo inmates:

1. Supply pattern of green forages during different seasons.
2. Alternate sources of green forage supply during scarcity caused by natural disasters like drought and flood.
3. Assured regular supply of good quality compounded feeds for different species.
4. Assured supply of buffen (buffalo meat) with long bones, other meats, rabbits and fishes for the carnivorous mammals and reptiles. Some carnivorous avian species also need flesh and small fishes.
5. Assured supply of wholesome drinking water, preferably running water or fresh and drinking water arrangement.
6. Arrangements in the enclosures for the supply of free choice mineral licks.
7. Supply of vitamins on short intervals and as per the requirements.

8. Supply of palatable medicated feed supplements for periodic deworming. Drug is also given in drinking water to avian species, rodents and lagomorphs.

Feeding Management of Zoo Animals in Groups

Feeding of animals in groups significantly reduces management activities but many times following problems need correction:

1. Aggressive animals : These animals do not allow others to eat in company. Some of these animals also spoil considerable amount of feeds.
2. Over eating and obesity occur in aggressive animals.
3. Selective feeding changes the nutritional composition of remaining feeds for the consumption of other animals.
4. Weak and recessive animals may suffer from the nutritional imbalance and resulting disorders.
5. For adequate supply, about 15-20% more feeds and fodder are offered.

The aggressive rogue animal should be either tethered in one corner of the paddock or should be isolated from individual feeding. This is essential for the maintenance of optimum health and good condition.

Feeding of the Tall and Long Necked Herbivores

Although long necked herbivores mammals like camels, giraffe and llamas easily adapt feeding on the mangers at much lower level than their height. However, in such arrangements, these animals require raising of head each time for deglutition after biting mouthful feeds. In order to provide comfortable feeding device in several zoos, tree leaves with twigs and lighter branches are offered on the towers at the level of the neck or a little above for providing natural feeding of browsing.

Feeding of the Common Browsing Herbivores

The wild members of caprine, antelopes and cervids are offered tree leaves intact on the branches. The branches of tree fodder are hanged on stands in the enclosures of the browsing herbivorous animals.

❑❑❑

7

Feeding of Suckling-starved Mammalian Neonates in Early Life

Introduction

Milk is the natural food of mammals in early life. The mammalian females have been evolved to provide the nutritional requirements of their infants in early life. The duration of nursing depends on the normal development of digestive system and food intake from other sources according to natural feed habits of the species.

Nursing Starvation

The non-availability of food by suckling in early life is known as nursing starvation.

Causes of Nursing Starvation

Followings are some of the observed causes of nursing starvation of mammalian neonatesm in early life. The incidence starts normally from the day of birth but can occur later also:

1. Occurrence of agalactia due to hormonal disturbances. It can be observed more in the first time young mothers.
2. Inflammation of the mammary glands (mastitis): The condition is very painful in the beginning and dam does not allow suckling. Although spoiled milk of captive mammalian female is removed with the use of a suckling device in captive animals of zoo but this can not be fed to the infants. Milk drawn from mastitis mammal generally contains variety of pathogenic microorganisms and/or their harmful metabolites. Milk of mastitis mammals is unfit for feeding and it should be disposed of aseptic after boiling or chemical treatment for the total eradication of the pathogenic organisms.
3. Abandoned infants: Incidence of abandoning infants is frequently found in the fields of standing cultivated crops around the forests inhabited by the wild animals, particularly the mammalian species. Incidence of abandoning infants is often observed in deer and antelopes living in the non-forest area of fallow land, waste land, degraded land, ranges and river basins. Author and the family of Colonel Bhagwan Raut reared an abandoned spotted deer fawn of few hours of age at Babugarh in Uttar Pradesh. The fawn was reared on bottle feeding of bovine and equine milk. The fawn was left free on the stud farm and it gradually started the sharing of concentrates and green forages with the mares.

Another incidence of rearing Chinkara fawn from first day of birth is from Rajasthan. The fawn was reared by breast feeding by a lactating lad of Bishnoi community devoted for the protection of wild animals and trees (specially in Khejri tree) in Rajasthan state of Bharat. Due to shrinkage of forests, incidence of straying and parturition of wild animals in the standing crops particularly the sugarcane crop is increasing. These abandoned fawns and cubs are initially reared by the farmers by bottle feeding the milk of cows, buffalo or goats. It is easier to rear the fawn alongwith other farm animals but feline cubs and pups of cervids are normally handed over to the nearest forest department or zoological garden.

4. Orphan infants: These infants are found crying due to hunger and lack of mother care. The dams either die at the time of delivery or killed by a predator or hunter. A few decades also when hunting was not strictly prohibited the tales of capture and rearing of cubs, fawn and pups can be reared in the villages around the forests. Recently, an elephant calf in Odisha has been reared by the forest department by bottle feeding of the bovine milk in early life.

Foods of Nursing-started Mammalian Infants

Mother's milk is the natural food of the mammalian infants right from the first day of the birth. Therefore, milk will be the food of nursing starved mammalian infants. The infant gradually accept their other natural food and processed foods according to species. The duration of milk feeding ranges from 4 weeks to 3 months in most of the terrestrial and arborial mammals normally required to be hand fed in a zoological garden or a guard but forest house. milk of cow and buffaloes is easily available at most of the places in the forest area reconstituted milk from the dry matter powder is fed.

Colostrum

The first milk drawn immediately after the parturition is called colostrum. The physico-chemical characteristics of the colostrum are significantly different than the milk of the same animals. The composition of colostrum changes at the fast rate to become normal milk in 3 to 7 days period in different species.

Properties of Colostrum

1. Colostrum contain higher quantity of total solids than the milk of the same animal.
2. It has higher protein concentration and high proportion of immuno-globulins, specially the protective gamma-globulim. Colostrum intake is more important in the neonates of the species lacking efficient placental transport of the immuno-globulins from the mother to foetus e.g. neonates of bovine, caprine, ovine, equine and canine. This passive immunity provided by the immuno-globulins in early life is essential for protection against several infectious diseases in early life until the system is developed in the body after few months of birth.
3. Colostrum is a concentrated source of digestible energy mostly in the form of fat.
4. Vitamin content is also much higher than the milk.
5. It has laxative effect and stimulates early expulsion of muconium (first faeces) and micturition. The later is also stimulated by the dam during licking the infant(s).
6. Lactose content is much less than the milk.
7. Colostrum is rich in many vitamins.

Composition of Colostrum

The composition of colostrum of some mammalian species is presented in Table 1.

Colostrum contains high concentration of gamma (γ) globulin, the major immuno-globulin. This kind of passive immunity through the feeding of colostrum is essential in the neonates of some species lacking placental transfer of immuno-globulins from the mother to foetus in the womb.

β_2-microglobulin is structurally similar to immuno-globulin is found in the colostrum and milk. It has been observed to be related with the immunity and histo-compatibility antigen system (Grove and Greenbird, 1982).

The Effect of Gastro-intestinal Secretions (Enzymes) on the Immuno-globulins of Colostrum and Milk

Since the antibodies are proteins, which are generally hydrolyzed in digestive system, the ability of neonates of some mammalian species is an unusual characteristic phenomenon. The duration of transportation of the colostral immuno-globulins through the tunica mucosa is functional only during the initial 1 to 2 days of birth in the bovine, equine, swine and canine. The duration is somewhat longer for 3 to 4 days in case of kids and lambs. Flow of gamma-globulin through thoracic duct is high during the 3 hours after first feeding of colostrum (Shannon and Lascelles, 1968). The value of γ-globulin falls gradually to stabilize at about 24 hours. At this stage passage of intact globulins is significantly decreased and digested as common protein in the small intestine.

Storage of Colostrum

Colostrum is highly sensitive to environment. It coagulates on heating. Only fresh colostrum can be stored by deep freezing. Therefore, wild animal parks and zoological garden should have working deep freezing arrangements. Surplus colostrum from a dam should be collected in a sterile receptacle, labelled properly for the species, date of collection, place of collection and quantity.

Alternate for Colostrum

Generally a combination of intravenous administration of mother serum and oral administration of a mixture of egg contents and castor oil are used. Mother serum provides passive immunity similar to the colostrum immuno-globulins. The mixture of egg contents and castor oil provides nutrients and also acts as a laxative and stimulates the expulsion of muconeum. Excretion of muconeum and urination assures the potency of two main excretory passages.

Milk

The composition of mammary secretion changes gradually to stabilize in the normal range of composition in 5-7 days in different species. From this stage it is called milk. There is great variation in nutritional composition of milk amongst the species. Therefore, it is important to know the nutritional composition of the milk. This helps in the standardization of easily available milk of cow and buffalo, and dry skimmed milk powder and water for the reconstitution of milk for different species of wild mammals in the zoos.

Composition of the Whole Milk of Domestic Animals

In first impression cows and buffaloes are considered dairy animals among the domesticated species, but in different countries goats, sheep, camel, mare and yak are also important milch species. Recently milking of Mithun *(Bos frontalis)* has also started in the north-east Bharatiya states after the introduction of tethering and semi-intensive feeding on the stalls.

Since, milk of domestic animals is the easily available source, it is important to know the composition of milk of different species and breeds of the domestic animals (Table 7.1).

Table 7.1 Composition of whole milk of domestic animals (%)

Species/ Breeds	Total solids (TS)	Milk fat	Protein	Lactose	Solid not fat	Ash
Cattle (Zebu or *Bos indicus*)						
Sahiwal	14.0	4.4	3.8	4.5	8.5	0.7
Gir	13.8	4.4	3.8	4.9	10.6	0.7
Tharparkar	14.4	4.2	3.5	4.5	10.2	0.7
Rathi	14.5	4.5	3.6	4.5	10.0	0.7
Sindhi	14.2	4.2	3.7	4.7	10.0	0.7
Gangatiri	13.8	4.4	3.7	4.8	9.4	0.7
Cattle (*Bos Taurus*)						
Holstein	11.5	3.5	3.2	4.1	8.0	0.7
Brown Swiss	14.4	4.8	3.6	4.2	9.9	0.7
Gurnesey	13.2	4.4	3.3	4.0	8.8	0.7
Jersey	14.5	5.1	3.8	3.9	9.4	0.7
Red Dane						
Buffaloes (*Bubalus bubalis*)						
Murrah	16.53	5.8	3.9	4.1	8.91	0.73
Nili-Ravi	18.34	6.7	4.17	4.78	9.4	0.92
Mehsana	17.96	6.7	4.36	4.83	91.	0.90
Bhadawari	17.0	9.6	3.91	4.50	9.6	0.84

Swamp	16.9	8.2	4.0	4.90	9.0	0.80
Goat						
Barbari	14.51	4.2	3.69	4.1	10.51	0.80
Jamunapari	12.36	3.7	3.49	4.25	9.1	0.79
Anglo Nubian	11.6	3.5	2.61	4.20	9.0	0.80
Saanen	11.6	3.6	3.4	4.1	8.9	0.80
Tegenberg	11.1	3.6	2.90	4.08	3.8	0.80
Sheep	13.2	8.2	6.2	4.9	12.0	0.90
Camel						
Bacterian	14.1	4.8	4.0	4.9	8.2	0.90
Dromedary	14.2	4.5	3.8	5.4	9.92	0.70
Llamoid						
Lhama		4.4				
Vicuna		4.4				
Mare	10.91	2.2	2.64	6.15	8.89	0.38

Composition of the Milk of Wild Animals

In order to select a milk of comparable gross composition of domestic animals or to reconstitute milk for the feeding of the nursing starved infants, it is important to know the gross composition of milk of different wild mammalian species.

The long list of milk composition (Table 7.2) of the wild mammals shows vast variation, particularly in the percentage of milk fat, total milk solids and lactose percentage. Milk composition of many difficult and aggressive species may not be representative average due to very small and random sample size of 1 to 5 females of any stage of lactation.

Table 7.2 Composition of whole milk of wild mammalian species (%)

Species	Total solids (TS)	Milk fat	Solid not fat	Protein	Lactose	Ash
Ant eater	32.0	20.0	12.0	11.0	0.2	0.8
Antelopes						
Black buck	23.0	9.0	14.0	9.0	4.5	0.5
Eland	22.3	10.0	12.3	7.0	4.0	1.3
Gazelle	35.5	19.0	16.5	12.0	3.0	1.4

Impala	35.2	20.0	15.2	11.0	2.4	1.4
Neelgai						
Pronghorn	24.3	13.0	11.3	6.0	2.4	1.4
Ass (donkey)	9.7	1.3	8.4	1.9	6.2	0.4
Bears						
Black bear	36.7	24.5	15.2	11.5	0.5	1.8
Grizzlt bear	36.5	22.4	14.1	11.0	0.6	1.4
Polar bear	45.7	33.0	12.7	11.0	0.3	1.4
Beaver	33.0	19.8	13.2	9.0	2.2	2.0
Bovines						
Bison	13.2	1.7	10.0	4.8	5.7	0.96
Buffaloes						
Indian	16.5	7.0	10.2	4.4	5.1	0.80
Swamp	17.6	8.2	10.1	4.0	4.9	0.80
African black	17.4	7.2	8.62	1.44	7.8	0.80
African red	17.6	7.6	9.11	3.30	4.55	0.80
Cattle						
Camelids						
Bactrian	11.45	4.8	8.25	3.90	5.8	0.85
Dromedary	11.94	4.6	8.25	2.54	4.71	0.79
Llama	13.1	4.4	8.95	4.2	5.9	0.76
Vicuna	12.5	4.6	8.95	3.70	7.40	0.76
Canines						
Dog	23.0	3.5	9.3	5.6	3.1	0.9
Fox	12.0	3.53	8.25	3.29	4.50	0.72
Hyena						
Jackal						
Wolf						
Caprines						
Cervids (Deer)						
Barking		4.8				
Dhaman		4.6				
Elk	17.5	6.7	12.4	6.4	4.7	1.0
Hog						
Sambhar		5.8				
Sikka		7.2				
spotted						

Composition of the Whole Milk of Different Mammalian Species

The available information on the composition of whole milk of different species are compiled in Table 7.3. The values of whole milk of certain species presented in Tables 7.2 and 7.3 are showing significant variations. This is due to availability of few samples (some times only one sample) from rare species. This aspect will require frequent revision.

Table 7.3 Composition of whole milk of different species (%)

Species	Fat	Protein	Lac-tose	Ash	References
Ant eater	20	11	0.3	0.8	Altman & Bittmer (1961)
Antelope					
Blackbuck	9	7	4.3	0.5	Author
Eland	10	6.7	3.9	1.3	Treus & Kravchenko, 1968
Gazelle	19.4	11.9	2.9	1.5	Ben Shaul, 1962
Impala	20.4	10.8	2.4	1.4	-do-
Pronghorn	13	6.1	4.0	1.3	Altmann & Bittmer, 1961
Baboon	5.0	1.6	7.3	0.3	Buss, 1968
Bear					
Black bear	24.5	14.5	0.4	1.8	Jenness et al., 1972
Grizzly bear	22.3	11.1	0.6	1.5	-do-
Polar bear	33.1	10.9	0.3	1.4	-do-
Beaver	19.8	9.0	2.2	2.0	Ben Shaul, 1962
Bison	1.7	4.8	5.7	0.9	Altmann & Bittmer, 1961
Buffaloes					
Chinese	12.6	6.0	3.7	0.9	Altmann & Bittmer, 1961
Egyptian	7.7	4.3	4.7	0.8	-do-
Philippine	10.4	5.9	4.3	0.8	-do-
Indian–Dairy					
Camel					
Bacterian	4.2	3.5	4.8	0.7	
Cat Cattle	7.1	10.1	4.2	0.5	Altmann & Bittmer, 1961
(*Bos taurus*)					
Ayrshire	4.9	3.6	4.7	0.7	Armstrong, 1959
Brown Swiss	4.0	3.6	5.0	0.7	

Guernsey	5.0	3.8	4.9	0.7	
Holstein	3.5	3.1	4.9	0.7	
Jersey	5.5	3.9	4.9	0.7	
Shorthorn	3.6	3.3	4.5	0.8	
Red steppes	3.9	3.3	4.6	0.8	
Kurgan	4.0	3.7	4.9	0.7	
Aulie-ata	3.6	2.9	-	0.2	
Taiga	4.1	-	4.7	0.8	
Latvian black	3.3		4.4	0.8	
Cattle, Zebu					
(*Bos indicus*)					
Hariana					
Sahiwal					
Gir					
Thaparkar					
Kankrej					
Cheetah	9.5	9.4	3.5	1.3	Ben Shaul, 1962
Chimpanzee	3.2	1.2	7.0	0.8	-do-
Chinchilla	12.5	8.0	1.7	1.0	Volcani et al., 1973
Collared	3.6	5.4	6.6	-	Sowls et al., 1961
Peccary					
Coyote	10.7	9.9	3.0	0.9	Ben Shaul, 1962
Deer	19.7	10.4	2.6	1.4	Spector, 1952
Spotted					
Hog					
Sikka					
Barking					
Sambhar					
Elk					
Dhaman					
Dog	9.5	9.3	3.1	1.2	Altmann & bittmer, 1961
Dolphin	41.5	10.9	1.1	0.7	-do-
Elephant	16.1	4.2	5.1	0.7	-do-
African					
Indian					
Fox	6.3	6.3	4.7	1.0	Young & Grant, 1931

Giraffe	13.5	5.8	3.4	0.9	Aschasselburg *et al.*, 1962
Goats	3.5	3.1	4.6	0.8	
Barbari					
Jamunapari					
Beetal					
Malabari					
Assamese					
Tellicheri					
Sirohi					
Gorilla	2.2	-	-	-	Ben Shaul, 1962
Guineapig	3.9	8.1	3.0	0.8	Nelson *et al.*, 1951
Hamster	12.6	9.0	3.4	1.4	Ben Shaul, 1962
Jedge jpg	10.1	7.2	2.0	2.3	-do-
Hippopotamus	4.5	-	4.4	0.1	Spector, 1956
Horse	1.6	2.4	6.1	0.5	
Human	4.3	1.4	6.9	0.2	
Jackal	10.5	10.0	3.0	1.2	Ben Shaul, 1962
Kangaroo	5.4	7.9	0.3	1.3	Bolliger & Pascoe, 1953
Leopard	6.5	11.1	4.2	0.8	
Lion	18.9	12.5	2.7	1.4	
Linx	6.2	10.2	4.5	0.8	
Mink	8.0	7.0	6.9	0.7	
Monkey					
Macaca mulatta	3.9	2.1	5.9	0.3	
Squirrel	5.1	3.5	6.3	0.3	
Moose	7.0	13.5	3.6	1.6	
Mouse	12.1	9.0	3.2	1.5	
Mule deer	1.8	2.0	5.5	0.5	
Musk ox	11.0	5.3	3.6	1.8	
Nutria	27.9	13.7	0.6	1.3	
Okapi	2.0	9.9	5.1	1.4	
Opossum	6.1	9.2	3.2	1.6	
Orangutan	3.5	1.4	6.0	0.2	
Otter	24.0	11.0	1.8	2.3	
Porcupine	13.2	12.4	1.8	2.3	

Puma	18.6	12.0	3.9	1.0
Hare				
Rabbit	12.2	10.4	1.8	2.0
Raccoon	3.5	8.0	6.6	1.0
Rat	13.0	9.7	3.2	1.4
Reindeer	20.9	10.0	2.5	1.4
Rhinoceros	-	1.5	6.12	0.3
Sea lion (California)	34.9	13.6	0.0	0.6
Seal				
Grey	53.2	11.2	2.6	0.7
Hart	42.6	10.4	-	0.8
Hooded	40.4	6.6	-	0.9
Sheep	10.4	6.8	3.7	0.9
Screw				
Short tail	6.5	11.0	3.2	0.8
Water	20.0	10.0	0.1	0.8
Squirrel	12.6	9.2	3.6	1.6
Swine (sow)	7.9	5.9	4.9	0.9
Tahr	-	9.8	3.0	1.3
Wolf (surohi)	9.6	9.2	3.4	1.6
Yak	-	5.2	4.6	-
Mithun Zebra	4.2	3.0	5.3	0.7

Use of Foster Mother

Use of foster mother for the rearing of the nursing starved or nursing deprived mammalian species is possible in the captive animals of zoo. Although, mammalian mothers are very sensitive in identifying their offsprings by marking them at birth as evident from the nursing behaviour of sheep and goats in the large flock and cows and buffaloes on the grazing land. There is great variation in the mothering behaviour of many mammalian species. Indeed good numbers of females are excellent mothers and happily adopt and nurse the starved infants.

Unusual Examples of Foster Mothers

There are many examples of inter-species nursing and rearing of deprived infants. Some breeds of dairy buffaloes allow suckling by any young buffalo calf of the herd. Heavy milk yielding cows are more liberal foster mother than the low milk yielding zebu cows. A spotted deer fawn abandoned by the dam near the boundary of the equine breeding stud was reared by Col. Bhagwan Raut and his daughter Mona on the bottle feeding of cow milk. Since the fawn was not exposed to out of the stud environment, it was allowed free movement within the walls of study. The fawn freely interacted with the workers, foals and mares. In this process good number of lactating mares allowed suckling. During the process of interaction the fawn learnt to eat the feeds offered to mares and the foals. At lunch time, it shared the Tiffin of the workers.

Another example was a lactating monkey that lost her baby within few days and adopted a pup. She breast fed the pup for few months and continued relationship even after drying.

The third example is a lady of Bishnoi community of Rajasthan. She reared an abandoned fawn of Chinkara on breast feeding in early life. The diet gradually included *bajra roti* mixed with milk or *chhanch*. The fawn was finally free to share concentrates and fodder of the farm animals.

Some Domestic Species Suitable for Foster Mother

Normally high milk yielding breeds of mammals more easily accept the infants of not their own species but also from other species. Dairy buffaloes, European breeds (*Bos taurus*) of cattle and European sows are easy foster mothers.

Beef cattle females on pasture are provided conditions for adopting early weaned calves. Beef cattle females are separated on another pasture after early weaning. This practice is used for reducing post partum breeding interval.

In kennels some selected bitches nurse the puppies of another bitch become a galactic and orphaned puppies. However, in many cases presence of bitch handler is essential and fostering is forced until gentle handling for willful acceptance of puppies. Once adopted, there is normally no discrimination between own and adopted puppies. A lactating bitch should nurse maximum 8 puppies including her own. Bitches with short litter are more suitable for use as foster mother.

Characteristics of Foster Mother

For ear marking foster mother(s) in a kennel, flock, herd or clan of the animals in captive conditions, following characteristics of a good mother should be observed:

1. The female should be a good lactating animal secreting more milk than the requirement of her own youngs.
2. It should not be aggressive against the youngs of fellow females or even the youngs of the other species.
3. It should be kind and affectionate.
4. Normally it should be approachable in size. However, there are exceptions of nursing puppies by a goat and vice-versa. There is also record of a monkey nursing an orphan street pup, a goat nursing a cattle calf and a lady of Rajasthan nursing an orphan Gazella fawn.

Frequency of Feeding

The number of bottle and pail or bucket feeding of nursing deprived infants depends on the species. Following pattern can be followed for the feeding of the infants of different species:

1. Infants of large herbivorous species are normally pail or bucket or bowl fed at about 12 hours interval. However, from the second week of life, the infants are offered compounded feed in mesh or crumbled form and thin stem leafy grasses or hay. With increasing age hunger stimulates eating of non-milk feeds from second to third week of age.
2. Infants of small herbivorous mammals are fed 3-4 times during the first two weeks of life and thereafter twice daily. Twice daily milk feeding can be followed even from the second week of birth.
3. Infants of omnivorous and carnivorous mammals are fed 4 times daily during the first two weeks. It is reduced to thrice daily during the next 2 weeks and thereafter twice daily. Infants of the omnivorous animals should be offered compounded feed in meshed or crumbled form.

Duration of Feeding the Nursing-starved Infants

The duration of milk feeding is normally 9 to 13 weeks. During this period infants learn to eat adequate amount of their normal feeds. However, some rare infants may require milk feeding for a little longer duration due to delayed learning of eating non-milk foods. In case of bucket or bowl feeding, mixing of small quantity of ground compound feed enhances consumption of compounded feeds (also grasses in herbivorous infants).

Health Care During Infant Rearing

1. Colostrum feeding should be arranged within 2-3 hours of parturition.
2. If colostrum is not available, alternate recipe should be used.
3. Milk of almost all mammals is deficient in iron content. Hence, parental iron preparations are injected as per standard schedule or oral preparations are drenched.
4. Booster dose of vitamins may be required.
5. Necessary vaccinations should be arranged.
6. Deworming schedule should be followed.
7. Exercise should be arranged as per the requirements of the species viz. calves, kids, lambs are left free in paddocks. Infants of primates are allowed exercise in enclosures containing branched trees protected under the wire mesh. Aquatic animals are provided shallow ponds. Cubs and pups are offered fresh lone bones.
8. As far as possible running drinking water should be provided.
9. There should be an adequate arrangement for protection against harsh climates.

Use of Eggs for the Feeding of Zoo Animal Infants

Eggs of different domestic birds are used in the diets of zoo animals under certain conditions:

1. In the diet of neonate mammals deprived of nursing/suckling the mother in early life.

2. In clinical cases and protein deficiency.
3. Raw egg white is used for the binding and expulsion of certain toxication.
4. Eggs are used for balancing the diets of carnivorous and omnivorous species in captive environment.

Gross composition of eggs of some common avian species is presented in Table 7.4.

Table 7.4 Gross composition of standard size eggs

Species	Weight (g)	Albumin (%)	Yolk (%)	Shell (%)
Fowl	58	56	32	12
Guinea fowl	40	52	35	13
Duck				
Goose	200	52	35	13
Turkey	85	56	32	12
Quail	10	48	32	20
Pigeon	15	74	18	8

Chemical (Nutritional) Composition of Common Edible Eggs

The chemical composition of edible parts of the eggs depicting the content of nutrients is important for balancing the composite diets of the carnivorous and omnivorous zoo inmates. Average values of protein, amino acids, lipids and vitamins are presented in Table 7.5.

Table 7.5 Average chemical/nutritional composition of eggs

Nutrients	Fowl	Guinea fowl	Duck	Goose	Turkey	Quail
Moisture	74	73	71	75	73	74
Dry matter	26	27	29	23	27	26
Protein	13	13	13	12	13	13
Lipids	12	12	12	12	12	11
Ash	1	1	1	1	1	1
Energy (Kcal/100g)	178	178	186	178	175	170

Nutritional composition of edible egg contents of different avian species is almost comparable. Amino acids and fatty acids are very important nutrients, and among these some constituents are dietary essential and must be supplied in the diet to meet the physiological requirements of the animals. Chicken eggs are used extensively because its production is much higher than any other avian species in the country. The amino acids and fatty acids composition of chicken eggs are presented in Table. Eggs of duck, goose and other avian species can be also fed. **Table.** Amino acids composition of eggs.

Appliances Used for the Artificial Feeding of the Suckling Starved Mammalian Infants

Different types of appliances are used for the feeding of milk and other fluid feeds for optimum nutrients supply to nursing starved infants. The selection of a feeding appliance depends on the size of animal, size of oral opening and requirement of the animal.

1. Use of common feeding bottle used for the feeding of human infants : The capacity of common feeding bottles for human infants is 100-125 ml. the shape of feeding bottle used in earlier days was boat-cum-spindle shape with both end open and capped with latex nipples (Fig. 7.1). It is always made of glass.

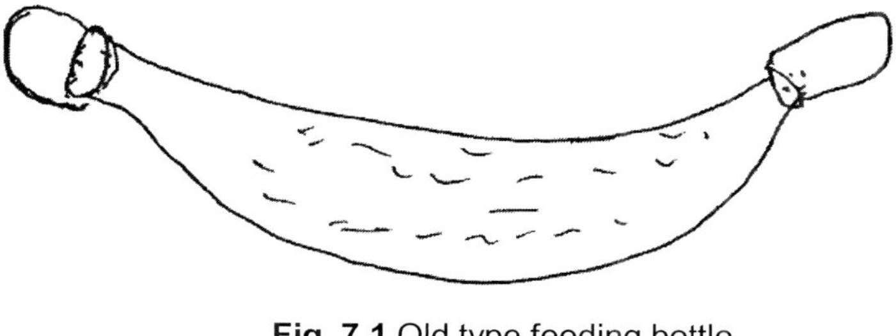

Fig. 7.1 Old type feeding bottle

2. Modern feeding bottles for human infants : The shape of modern feeding bottle is now cylindrical. It may be plan or graduated and marked in ounce (oz) or millilitres (ml). It contains only one wide mouth to be capped with a larger latex cap (Fig. 7.2), imitating the shape of human nipple. It is made of glass, stainless steel, aluminium alloy or good quality plastic. Sterilization of bottle is easy. Fig. 7.2 Cylindrical feeding bottles.

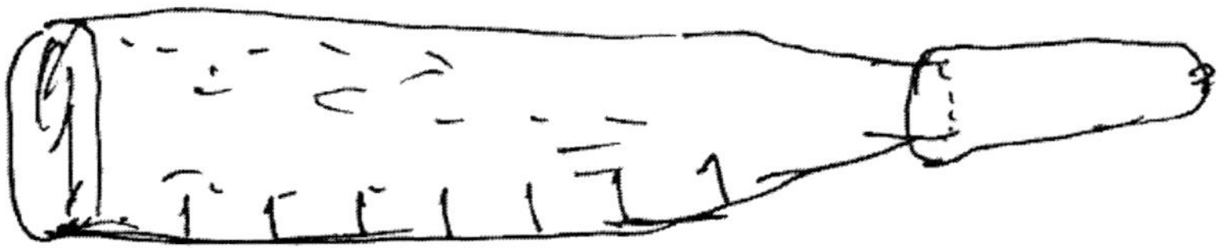

Fig. 7.2 Graduated feeding bottle

Cleaning of bottles : The feeding bottles should be immediately washed with a mild detergent, rinsed with clean water and dried at a clean place or in the oven.

3. Spoon feeding : Special spoon fitted with narrow tube (Fig.7.3) is used for the feeding of mammalian species of small size with narrow oral opening.
4. Cotton feeding : The tiny starved infants of some very small mammals are fed by dropping milk from the milk soaked sterilized cotton wool.

❑❑❑

8

Study Tour to Wildlife Reserve Forest, Zoo and Wildlife Institute

Introduction

The teaching will be complete only on the observation of feeding behaviour of the wild animals in situ and captive animals in zoo. The visits to wildlife reserves should not be a casual visit for sight seeing and recreation but it should be an educational tour of 4 to 6 or more working days depending on the accessible area and types of wild animal species in the sanctuary, park of reserve. The duration of observations of feed preparation, quantity allotment, systems of feed offering, watering, removal of the droppings, cleaning of the feeders, waterers and enclosures and disposal of the wastes in a zoo should be 2-3 working days. An experienced person responsible for the feeding of zoo inmates and zoo veterinarians should guide the students on the spot observations.

Wildlife Reserve Forests

The wildlife reserve forests are known by different names. Sometimes it is also named on a single important or threatened species or a class of animals like tiger reserve, lion safari, bird sanctuary, etc. although other wild animals are also found and protected.

Preparations Before Visiting a Wildlife Reserve

A visit to wildlife reserve for study requires following preparations:

1. The students and teachers should collect basic information about the herbage cover, climate and wild animal species in the forest.
2. Each person must have a gum boot and clothes should preferably be dull green to dull brown. Also, put a cap.
3. Each person should carry a bag on his/her back. The bag should contain a good torch, a knife, drinking water bottle (2 litres), cold drink, biscuits, a towel, paper napkins and glucose, etc. in top pocket there should be a note book and pen.
4. An umbrella or a raincoat may be needed in wet season.
5. Winter cloth should be sweaters and pull over or jacket but not long coat and suits.
6. A strong and hard stick fitted with sharp spike on the distal end.
7. A strong and smooth rope of 8-10 mm diameter and 8-10 m length.
8. Exploration deep in the forest should not be taken alone. There should be atleast three persons in the team.
9. A compass and a map showing layout and common herding places of different species of animals.

10. It will be always in the interest of the visitors to take the help of an experienced and trained guide of the forest. The guide should be familiar with the movement pattern and vocalization of different species.

11. For movement inside the forest, facilities provided by the jungle safari should be used. Motor vehicles should be used for movement on the forest roads. For the exploration of deep forest the footpaths formed by regular movements of different wild animal species should be followed.

12. An experienced jungle guide knows to greater extent the relationship among the arboreal, terrestrial and aquatic species. This will be helpful for observation of food preference, feeding habits and relationship among the species for food sharing.

13. For the study of feeding of the nocturnal animals, the students and teacher should take complete rest during the daytime.

14. If possible, an experienced and licensed hunter with licensed fire arm should be hired for the observations in deep forest used for shelter by canines, felines and reptiles, etc.

15. While entering into the forest, each one is required to reach the instructions displayed eligibly at the entrance of the wildlife sanctuaries. Specific instructions with arrow directions are also displayed boldly at road bifurcations and multiple branching.

16. One must ensure that mobile phone is charged and has enough balance (if prepare).

17. Important phone numbers of forest office, entrance point and other help points must be carried safe.

18. Loud noise and display of music instruments are strictly prohibited.

19. Visitors are not allowed to offer any kind of food and drinks to wild animals.

20. There should be a good first-aid box. It should also contain a tourniquet for stopping blood circulation, if essential.

21. A camera with adequate zoom is needed. Movie camera is useful for recording food preference, bites, chewing and swallowing, etc. it is also used for recording predation technique of different

carnivorous species. Zoom camera helps the recording of wild animals averse for the presence of humans.

22. Information should also be gathered from the forest personnel regarding presence and location of bee hives in the forest.
23. Study tour should not be made adventure tour.

Motor Vehicle Suitable for Jungle Safari

A motor vehicle for jungle safari should have following characteristics and facilities:

1. It should be four wheels driven hard body jeep.
2. Half body should be covered and posterior half should be open.
3. Wild glass, windows and open part should be protected with strong metallic bars for protection from the felines, canines, elephants, wild buffaloes, primates and other dangerous animals.
4. Ground cleaning space should be high.
5. Fuel tank should be capacious and strong to bear rock strike, if any.
6. The vehicle should be fitted with a hook for inserting a chain, if toeing is required.

Closing of Camp in the Forest

If group has camped in the jungle for study, it must be in the knowledge of the forest personnel responsible for the management. Prior written permission should be obtained. Observations of the feeding of nocturnal animals should be recorded carefully.

At the end of camp, the place must be cleaned and waste materials should be disposed of at a place made for it. If camp is at an isolated place, all the waste materials should be completely burnt. The first must be extinguished before living the site. The forest personnel should be informed before leaving and thanked for the facilities and cooperation provided for the study.

Things Carried from the Forest for Laboratory Study

Adequate number of containers, markers and sealing materials should be carried for the collection of food and faecal samples.

Following precautions should be taken during collection and packaging:

1. The herbage sample should contain leaves, stem, inflorescence and fruits as per the availability.
2. Green samples should not be kept in closed containers, because sweating is a continuous process of green herbage. This moisture should continuously evaporate. Accumulation of moisture often causes rotting and spoils the phenotype due to which identification is not possible.
3. Samples of green herbages are tied and tagged in small bundles. The tag contains date and time of collection, place of collection and the animal eating the herbage.
4. Faecal droppings are collected in a plastic pan. A fraction is placed in a stoppered wide mouth glass bottle and treated with small quantity of sulphuric acid (known volume) for binding faecal nitrogen and stopping enzyme activities. The other part is sun dried or air dried (if possible) and then put in a polyethylene bag, tied and labeled properly for further analysis in laboratory.

Identification of Herbage and Analysis of the Biological Samples of Nutritional Importance

1. Undamaged samples containing leaves and other parts (inflorescence, fruits, roots), if available, should be sent to botany department link for identification.
2. Identified plant should be processed and preserved in a suitable herbarium record book. Important characteristics and uses should be recorded.
3. Dried fruits and kernels are preserved in labelled wide mouth stoppered transparent bottles.
4. A record book should contain complete information of the samples comprising of place and date of collection.

Study Tour to Zoo(s)

For understanding the actual feeding practice of animals in a zoo, the students should be shown at least one big zoo at nearest place from the veterinary college. Before visiting a zoo for the study of food preparation and feeding some basic information should be requested from the Director of the zoo.

Points to be Considered for the Selection of Zoo for Study Tour

1. As far as possible zoo should be nearer to college.
2. The zoo should house important and raise species of territorial, arborial and aquatic animals.
3. There should be representatives of herbivorous, carnivorous and omnivorous animals.
4. There should be representatives of mammals, reptiles and avian species normally not accessible to most of the people.
5. There should be also some nocturnal and burrow making animal species.

Preparations for Study Tour to Zoo

Following preparations are required by the students before a study tour to zoo:

1. Location and distance of zoo.
2. Condition of the road.
3. Availability of hostel, guest house or hotels for boarding and lodging.
4. Classes and species of wild and rare animals in the zoo.
5. Record book, pen and pencil, etc.
6. Dress as per visit to jungle safari.
7. Articles like camera, movie camera, gum boot and others as per the season and climate.

Observations to be Recorded Regarding the Feeding of Zoo Animals

1. Raw foods offered to different species.
2. Processed foods offered to different species.
3. Methods of preparation of special foods.

4. Time of feeding to different species.
5. Frequency of feeding to different species.
6. Frequency and method of feeding vitamins and other additives, if any.
7. Cleaning of feeders and waterers.
8. Sequence of offering different feeds in case more than one kind of feed is offered.
9. Approximate time taken by different species for feed intake.
10. Inspection of animals during feed. This is important for observing the soundness of the animals. Unhealthy/sick animals avoid feed intake either due to loss of appetite or inability to eat due to injury or inflammation of the oral cavity.
11. Isolation of sick animal to sick ward.

Preparation of Special Diets for the Sick Animals

The special diets include soup, slurry, gruel, pudding, juice and mash, etc. Some carnivorous and omnivorous animals are also fed fruits, milk, eggs and curdm etc. as per the requirement.

Feeding of Pregnant

Pregnant females are separated from the group on appropriate time decided for the different species. This is normally practiced for the large animals housed in groups. The animals are housed in maternity home and fed special diets recommended for feeding during late pregnancy and lactation period.

The tour terminates with thanks to zoo personnel.

Study Tour to Wildlife Institute

The wildlife Institute of India is situated in the campus of the Indian Forest Research Institute, Dehradun in Uttrakhand. Main activities of the Institute are the teaching and training of graduates and post graduates on wildlife management in situ and in zoo. Teaching is organized through the subject-matter divisions.

❑❑❑

9

Harmful Substances in Feedstuffs

Introduction

The natural constituent(s) in feed ingredients producing non-toxic or toxic harmful effect on the body are known as anti-nutritional factors. Almost all proteinous feeds of plant origin contain one or more anti-nutritional constituents.

Characteristics of Harmful Substances

Different kinds of harmful substances are found even in the common feed ingredients of poultry and other farm animals. The chemical composition and properties of these substances are highly variable and may be acidic, alkaline or neutral in nature.

1. These substances have adverse effects of voluntary intake, digestibility, absorption and metabolism.
2. Some factors produce anti-nutritional effects and in some feeds their metabolites produce harmful or even toxic effects.
3. Many anti-nutritional factors are unstable and either destroyed or inactivated by simple processing techniques like drying, boiling, roasting, pressure cooking, soaking and fermentation, etc.
4. A few factors turn toxic during digestion due to change in chemical composition viz., feed nitrates are reduced in nitrites which are toxic and may be fatal on crossing threshold. The nitrites bind with the haemoglobin of erythrocytes and convert ferrous form of iron in haemoglobin to ferric form in brownish methaemoglobin. The methaemoglobin is not capable of transporting oxygen to different tissues causing anoxia and death. Scope of nitrate/nitrite poisoning in poultry is difficult from feed sources.

Different Kinds of Harmful Substances in Feeds

Different kinds of anti-nutrient constituents of the various feed stuffs and also the adulterants of feeds like mixing the argemone seeds with rape seed-mustard have been identified and listed in Table 9.1.

Table 9.1 Harmful substances in conventional and non-conventional feeds

S.No.	Harmful factors	Feed sources
1.	Protease inhibitors (e.g. trypsin inhibitors)	Leguminous seeds - soyabeans, clusterbean seeds, field beans, peas
2.	Phenols	
	a) Gossypol	Cotton seed and cotton seed cake
	b) Tannins	Sorghum, mustard, rapeseed cake, salseed meal, mango seed kernel, tamarind seed, babool seed, black berry (jamun) seed, etc.

3.	Phytates	All feeds of plant origin.
4.	Oxalates	Sesame seed meal, many plant and animal feeds
5.	Nimbidins	Neem seed and neem seed meal
6.	Nitrates and nitrites	Immature plants, chemical contami nation
7.	Non-starch polysaccharides (NSPs)	Cereal grains, brans and vegetable proteins
8.	Mimosine	Leucaena (koobabul/subabul) leaf meal
9.	Glycosides	
	a) Cyanogenic	Linseed meal, tapioca root
	b) Glucosinolates	Mustard-rapeseed meal
	c) Oestrogens	Soyabean seed, lucerne leaf meal
	d) Saponins	Soyabean meal, lucerne leaf meal, mahua seed meal
10.	Haemagglutitins or lectins	Soyabean, kidney bean, castor beans, cluster bean meal
11.	Erucic acid	Mustard rape seed
12.	Argemone	Adultrant in mustard rape seed meal
13.	Antivitamin factors	
	a) Antivitamin A	Soyabean seed (Lipoxygenase enzyme)
	b) Antivitamin D	Soyabeans
	c) Antivitamin E	Kidney bean
	d) Antivitamin K	Dicumarol (false vitamin K synthesis) in sweet clover
	e) Antivitamin B_1 or antithiamine	Linseed meal
	f) Antipyridoxine	Linseed (linamarin)

Harmful Effects of Various Harmful Substances

The information about various anti-nutritional factors naturally occurring as constituents of many common feed resources and their deleterious effects on the health and production of poultry are important. These information are used for the selection of suitable feedstuffs and also application of suitable treatment for the inactivation/detoxification of such feed. Deleterious effects of different anti-nutritional factors on the health and production of poultry birds need attention during selection of feeds and formulation of compounded diets.

1. Protease inhibitors (trypsin inhibitors)

These are harmful constituents are present in many vegetable foods. So far, about six protease inhibitors have been found. The important ones are the Bowman-Birk chymotrypsin inhibitors and the Kunitz antitrypin factor. Protease inhibitors reduce availability of protein by reducing digestion and absorption. In an attempt to neutralize the harmful effect of protease inhibitors, the pancreas attempts to increase protease secretion that results in the hypertrophy of the pancreas. This reaction is harmful for health.

Protease inhibitors are also proteinous and heat labile and destroyed by heat treatment of foods. Both dry and moist heat treatments are effective. The potent sources of protease inhibitors are seeds of soyabean, cluster bean, jack bean and many leguminous seeds.

Protease inhibitors reduce digestibility of protein causing deficiency of amino acids resulting in reduced growth and egg production. Requirement of methionine is increased due to endogenous losses.

Common methods of destruction of protease inhibitors in feed ingredients are toasting, autoclaving or pressure flowing hot steam through the feeds.

2. Phenolic compounds in feeds

Two common phenolic compounds in feeds of plant origin are gossypol and tannins.

a) **Gossypol** : It is a toxic phenolic compound of yellow colour found in cotton seeds. The content varies in different varieties and may range from 0.03-2.0% in dry matter. It is an aldehyde in chemical property. Gossypol is anti-oxidant and inhibits polymerization reactions. Total gossypol in cotton seed/cotton seed cake is present in bound and free forms and the later causes toxic effects. The proportion of free gossypol is greater but variable and may be upto 70% of the total gossypol. The concentration of gossypol in cotton seed meals depends on the method used for oil extraction. Free gossypol content in hydraulic pressed, screw-pressed, solvent extracted and pre-pressed solvent extracted cotton seed meals may be in range of 0.4-1.0%, 0.2-0.5%, 0.2-0.7% and 0.2-0.3% on dry matter basis, respectively. During the process of oil extraction greater proportion of free gossypol binds with protein to form almost undegradable protein complex. This has negative effect on protein digestibility and lysine availability.

Incorporation of cotton seed meals for protein supply in composite poultry feeds should not be more than 10% to limit the concentration of free gossypol below 0.1% which is considered the tolerance level for poultry. For the neutralization of higher gossypol content in compounded feeds, ferrous sulphate can be mixed. The amount of ferrous sulphate may be upto 4 times of gossypol.

Concentration of more than 0.1% produces adverse effects on the performance of health of poultry birds. Prolonged use of cotton seed meal in the diets of poultry may be fatal. The clinical symptoms in growing chicks are loss of appetite, laboured breathing, cardiac disorders and decreased growth rate. In laying hens, even small quantity causes greenish discolouration of egg yolk. Fall in oxygen transportation capacity of red blood cells results in hypoxia of tissues and associated pathological changes.

b) **Tannins** : These are complete polyphenolic compounds and constituents of many feeds of plant origin, seeds, cereal grains and extractions. The two main forms of tannins in feeds are the condensed tannins and hydrolysable tannins. Small quantity of tannins may be beneficial but considerable concentration is antinutritional because tannins bind proteins and carbohydrates and render them indigestible. These also inhibit the activities of digestive enzymes (protease, amylase and lipase, etc). more than 0.5% tannins in the composite diets of poultry reduces digestibility of proteins and carbohydrates and rate of decrease is more or less proportional to concentration of tannins but beyond 4% level may be even fatal due to drastic fall in feed intake and availability of nutrients from such feeds. Lower tannin content in feeds decreases availability of nutrients resulting in lowered growth rate in chicks and fatal in egg production of layers.

Tannins containing common feeds of poultry are sorghum, milo, rape seed mustard seed cake and Lucerne leaf meal. Non-conventional feeds like deoiled sal seed meal, mango seed kernel, tamarind seed, mahua seed kernel cake. Tannins content in these feeds are very high and require laborious and expensive technologies for nutritional improvement. Therefore, use of nonconventional feeds containing more than 2-3% tannins can not be recommended. Total concentration of tannins should not exceed 0.5% of dry matter. Higher tannins content in diets may not have significant adverse effect on voluntary feed intake but availability of protein and energy decreases. The effects are lowered growth performance of chicks and fall in egg production.

3. Glycosides

These are complete carbohydrates which may ester condensation products containing alcohol, phenol or sugars and lignosaccharides. These are generally antinutritional for the animals. The glycosides present naturally in the feeds of plant sources are cyanogens, saponins, glucosinolates and oestrogenic substances.

a) **Cyanogenic glucosides** : Instant cyanogenic glucosides are not deleterious. Rupture of cells during grinding in gizzard releases glucosidase enzymes that hydrolyze cyanogenic glucosides and highly toxic hydrocyanic acid (HCN) is released.

b) **HCN is highly toxic** and inhibits the cytochrome oxidase which regulates enzyme action which is responsible for the cell respiration. The HCN is a fatal toxin and death is spontaneous in few seconds. Damaged or bruised tapioca (cassava) root is a potent source of cyanogenic glucosides. For use in poultry feeds, tapioca root should be boiled, water is drained out and boiled roots are dried and ground for feeding.

c) **Saponins :** These are toxic glycosides that decrease surface tension and form foam with proteins and sterols. Saponins decrease the availability of cholesterol by forming complex compounds which are eliminated in excreta. Level of cholesterol in blood and liver falls. Leguminous leaf meal prepared from Lucerne berseem and other clovers contain substantial amount of saponin and incorporation of high level (say 20% or more) or higher than 0.37% saponin content from leaf meals and other sources depressed body weight gin in chicks. In contrast with blood, saponins cause haemolysis and change cell permeability. Respiration rate is increased in affected birds. Egg production decreased in laying eggs.

d) **Phytoestrogens :** The phytoestrogen more concerned with poultry nutrition is an isoflavone called genistein present in soyabean seeds. The factor is active in raw soyabeans and inactivated on heat treatment. Genistein enhanced absorption and deposition of excess amount of several minerals like calcium, phosphorus and manganese in bones and zinc content in liver and bones. Phytoestrogens ae not fat soluble substances and residue left in soyabean meal after solvent extraction is inadequate to have any appreciable effect on metabolism. Growth is depressed and feed utilization efficiency is reduced.

e) **Glucosinolates or thioglucosinolates or goitrogens** : These are complex organic compounds responsible for reducing the availability of iodine and development of goiter for compensating the requirement of thyroid hormones. Glucosinolates or thioglucosinolates present in rape seed, mustard seed meal are hydrolyzed to yield goitrogenic compounds, 2-OH-3 butanyl isothiocyanate and 5-vinyloxazolidinine-2-thionegoitroin. These suppress iodine uptake resulting in goiter development. The other harmful effects are poor growth, low feed conversion efficiency, decreased egg production and haemorrhages and fatty changes in liver.

4. Erucic acid

It is polyenoic unsaturated fatty acid responsible for pungent taste o rape seed-mustard seed oil. Nominal residue is present in solvent extracted meals. Poultry feeds containing less than 0.5% erucic acid has no adverse effect on voluntary intake and performance of birds. The harmful effect has been almost removed due to extensive production of solvent extracted cakes. Use of high proportion of expeller pressed rape seed-mustard seed cake in poultry feeds will reduce voluntary feed intake, poor growth response and decreased feed conversion efficiency. Now in many countries low erucic acid or no erucic acid rape-mustard seeds (e.g. carola seed) have been developed by genetic manipulation.

5. Phytases (salt of phytic acid)

These are organic compounds of high molecular weight formed from the estrification of a cyclic alcohol inositol with six phosphate molecules. In addition to phosphorus other dietary essential minerals also bind with complex phytate (phytin) molecules which are constituents of plants. The concentration of phtates is generally high in protein rich feeds of plant origin. Simple stomached animals including poultry do not produce sufficient quantity of enzyme phytatase, necessary for the liberation of phosphorus and other minerals chelated in the feed. The other minerals in phytate molecules are calcium, magnesium and trace elements manganese and zinc. The balancing of these minerals in poultry feeds requires special attention for ensuing supply of these minerals. The problem is resolved by either increasing the concentration of these minerals by mixing inorganic salts of higher availability or mixing adequate quantity of exogenous phytase enzyme in compounded feeds. Six molecules of phosphate are chelated with the phytic acid and calculation of phosphorus supply only on the basis of chemical composition is highly misguiding and results in phosphorus deficiency although concentration in feeds is adequate. Phytates are also responsible for decreasing the availability of amino acids and carbohydrates.

6. Non-starch polysaccharides (NSPs)

These are constituents of feeds of plant origin. The non-starch polysaccharides are cellulose and hemicellulose present in bread and these are not digested in the birds due to non-availability of enzymes required for hydrolysis into digestible and absorbable forms. Cellulose, a fibrillar polysaccharide is a polymer of glucose molecules united by 1,4-β-bonds. Hemicelluloses and pectins constitute the matrix of cell wall complexed with lignin. Composition of hemicelluloses is complex and yet less defined. The pectin substances are polymers of galacturonic acid methyl ester. In addition to these, a group of soluble NSPs like β-glucans, arabinoxylan, arabinogalactans, glactomannans, glacturananans, xyloglucans and rhamnogalacturonans are harmful for the poultry. The contents of some harmful NSPs in common feeds are presented in Table 9.2.

Table 9.2 Non-starch polysaccharides (NSPs) in some common feeds

Sl.	Non-starch polysaccharide	Poultry feed ingredient
1.	Arabinoxylans	Maize, wheat
2	Arabinogalactans	Mustard seed, rape seed
3	β-Glucans	Barley, oats
4	Galactomannans	Cluster bean seed
5	Galactoarabinans	Soyabean seed
6	Galacturananans	Soyabean seed
7	Rhamnogalacturonans	Lupin seeds

7. Argemone (an adulterant in rapeseed-mustard seed)

The prickly poppy is a weed and its seeds are easily mixed with black rape seed-mustard seed and often used for adulteration of rape-mustard seed. It contains a toxin.

8. Mimosine

It is a harmful protein present in subabul (earlier and truly koobabul, *Leucaena leucocephala*) and binds with iodine causing iodine deficiency and decrease in level of thyroid hormones. This causes disturbances in energy and minerals (calcium and iodine) metabolism. The symptoms are reduction in growth rate of chicks, loss of body weight in adults, thinness of egg shell in layers, reproduction insufficiency or even failure and enlargement of thyroid gland (goiter). Leucaena leaf meal incorporation in poultry feeds for protein and carotenoids supply should not be recommended.

9. Nimbidn

Neem seed kernel cake is a rich source of protein but its feed value is significantly reduced due to presence of harmful constituents known as nimbidins. The three anti-nutritional (bitter) factors of neem seed are nimbine, nimbinin and nimbidine. Mixing of neem seed kernel cake in poultry feeds reduces voluntary feed intake resulting in decreased supply of protein, energy and other nutrients precipitating in lowered growth rate and egg production, damage of vital organs and death on prolonged feeding.

10. Anti-vitamins

Certain feeds contain substances that either inactivate some vitamins or reduce their potency:

a) **Antivitamin A** : An enzyme lipoxygenase present in raw soyabean seeds oxidases carotenoids (the precursors of vitamin A) in mixed feeds and reduces the availability of vitamin A resulting in occurrence of vitamin A deficiency symptoms (see vitamin A), the dietary requirement of performed vitamin A increases.

b) **Antivitamin D** : It is also present in raw soyabean seeds and increases the dietary requirement of vitamin D_3 in poultry feeds for optimum functions. The deficiency symptoms are bone deformities and thinness of egg shells as observed in vitamin D deficiency.

c) **Antivitamin E** : Antivitamin E factor is found in raw kidney bean (*Phaseolus vulgaris*). Inclusion of raw kidney bean in the diets of poultry causes development of reproductive disorders. However, problem is solved by supplementation of higher quantity of vitamin E. Probably antivitamin E factor in kidney beans does not interfere in the action of supplemented vitamin E which is higher due to non-availability of constituent vitamin E in feed ingedients.

d) **Antivitamin K** : A factor present in sweet clover (*Melilotus albus*) known as coumarins which are converted to dicoumbarol by fungi like Aspergillus species infestation during the production of leaf meal in bad weather. Dicoumarol decreases the synthesis of prothrombin in blood necessary for clotting and control of bleeding. Contamination of feeds with dicoumarol increases the requirement of vitamin K in compounded poultry feeds.

e) **Antivitamin B_6 or antipyridoxine factor :** A compound linatine present in linseed (flax seed) meal is a peptide composed of 1-amino D praline and glutamic acid. It reduces the potency of pyridoxine and produces deficiency. The deficiency symptoms are lowered appetite, reduced growth rate, encephalomalacia and chondrodystrophy. The nervous damage is exhibited by jerking movement of legs and wings. The affected chicks run uncontrolled with flapping sings and die. Sometimes affected birds roll on back with legs upwards. There may be paddling in some patients, inappetance, loss of body weight, lowered egg production and death.

f) **Antivitamin B_1 or antithiamian factor :** An enzymic thiaminase in bracken fern (*Pteridium equilibrium*) and raw fish meal. Thiamin activities of feeds are destroyed by mixing raw fish meal or bracken fern leaf meal in the diets of poultry.

Methods of Inactivation, Destruction, Neutralization and Extraction of Harmful Substances in Feeds

In order to improve the nutritive and feeding values of feed ingredients various methods have been developed and standardized for practical uses by the poultry farmers and commercial feed manufacturing companies. Some useful methods are summarized in Table 9.3.

Table 9.3 Methods of inactivation, neutralization and removal of harmful factors in feed ingredients

No.	Anti-nutrients in feeds	Method(s) of treatment
1.	Protease inhibitors	Dry or moist heat treatments like roasting and cooking are effective treatments.
2	Haemagglutinins	Mustard seed, rape seed
3.	Saponins	
4.	Cyanogens	Sun drying giving full exposure by several turning of cassava tuber chips/small pieces
5	Oestrogenic substances	Heat treatment
6	Glucosinolates	Solvent extracted rape seed-mus tard seed meal is used below 10% to keep the level of glucosinolates below 0.6% in complete feeds.
7.	Erucic acid	
8.	Phytates	Phytase enzymes of fungal sources are used as effective feed supple ment.
9.	Gossypol	Use of cotton seed meal is avoided in poultry feeds. In shortage less than 5% is mixed in composite diets.

10.	Tannins	Small quantity of tannins containing feeds are mixed to keep the level of tannins below 0.2% in complete feeds.
11.	Argemone	Argemone contaminated feeds are not used.
12.	Mimosine	Leucaena (subabool) leaf meal should not be used.
13.	Nimbidine	Ammoniation is claimed effective. Not yet widely used.
14.	Non-starch polysaccharides	Some commercial mixtures of poly enzymes are claimed effective.
15.	Antivitamin A	Heat treatment of soybean seeds.
16.	Antivitamin D	Heat treatment of soyabean seeds.
17.	Antivitamin E	Kidney bean should not be used for poultry feeding.
18	Antivitamin K	Sweet clover leaf meal should not be used in poultry feeds.
19.	Antivitamin B_6 (Linatine)	Supplementation of vitamin B_6 (pyri doxine) is essential for use of linseed meal in poultry diet.
20.	Antivitamin B_1	Thiaminase containing fish meal should not be used in poultry feeds for balancing essential amino acids.

❑❑❑

10

Flying is No Escape:
Migratory Birds and Climate Change

According to Hans Verolme, Director of World Wildlife Fund (WWF) Global Climate Change Programme, 'birds have long been used as indicators of environmental change' and a recent global status report entitled, Birds Species and Climate Change (2006), indicated that birds are 'the quintessential canaries in the coal mine' when it comes to climate change. So, it is of particular concern that at present, the prognosis for bird species – whether they are migratory, mountain, island, wetland, arctic, Antarctic or seabirds – it most dreadful. The report clearly assembles scientific evidence which demonstrates a 'trend towards a major bird extinction from global warming'.

The May, 2008, International Union for the Conservation of the Nature (IUCN) assessment concluded that 'climate change – and even some attempts to tackle it – are pushing one in eight species of birds towards extinction. In the past year alone, 26 of the 1226 species on their 'Red List' of threatened bird species became more endangered while only 2 species improved in status.

The Bird Species and Climate Change (2006) report warns that extinction rates 'could be as high as 38 per cent in Europe and 72 per cent in northeastern Australia, if global warming exceeds 2°C above the pre-industrial levels (currently it is 0.8°C above)'. Unfortunately, the current approach to bird conservation which focuses on protecting specific and limited areas containing high bird diversity will inevitably fail, simply because climate change will force birds to shift into unprotected zones as they desperately try to cope with an ever warming planet and the shifts this brings to their habitats. In the United States bird populations have also shrunk, and nearly a third of the bird species living in the eastern Midwest and Great Lakes areas could be lost in other parts of the world, the situation is just as precarious, it not worse.

In the Australian north-eastern wet tropics, almost three quarters of the rainforest birds are at risk of disappearing. Elsewhere on that continent, increase severe droughts accompanied forest fires have decimated the populations of Australian Mallee Emuwren (Stipiturus mallee). Their numbers have not plummeted and the largest population now numbers just 100 and is constrained to a 100 square kilometer plot of land. The IUCN warns that a single forest fire could have dramatic consequences and has listed the species as endangered. The plight of the Australian Mallee Emuwren is not unique. In fat, many regions on which birds depend may soon become unsuitable due to climate change. Island and mountain birds may simply have nowhere to go and changes may make it impossible for annual migrations to take place.

A 2007 article by Alister Doyle, 'Migratory Birds and Whales Confused by Warming' revealed that a 'warmer climate disrupts the biological clocks of migratory species including bats, dolphins, antelopes or turtles' these animals are now the most visible warning signs (or) indicators signaling the dramatic changes to our eco systems caused in parts by climate change. Scientists warn in North America, 'Spring migration is occurring earlier and fall migration later in many species. For example, 25 migratory bird species are arriving in Manitola Canada earlier then they did 63 years ago". As changes between seasons continue to become less clear, many birds are mistiming their migratory pattern. These shifts make them quite vulnerable to heat waves, droughts or cold snaps.

Of particular concern is the fact that some bird populations are abandoning their migrations altogether. For instance, cranes are starting to spend the winter in Germany rather than fly sough in Spain or Portugal. Birds exhibiting their behaviour risk remaining in regions that can potentially be too cold for them to survive. In such cases, a single severe winter event could decimate entire populations.

Furthermore, migratory birds are particularly vulnerable as they depend heavily upon separate breeding, wintering and stop-over sites. Changes to any one of the habitats can put them at risk. The report, 'Bird Species and Climate Change' points out that climate change is pushing birds out of synchrony with key elements of their ecosystems. The fact that migratory birds are characteristically very prompt and sensitive responders to any fluctuations in climate leaves them particularly vulnerable. Species of birds that rely on limited areas for their breeding, to which they may travel very long distances, may be pushed out of existence in a large scale much sooner than previously anticipated, while some bird populations are already facing drastic reductions in their numbers. In fact, scientists have found declines of upto 90 per cent in some bird populations, as well as total and unprecedented reproductive failure in others.

With the increase in temperature in the Arctic region, for example, 'forests could take over from tundra, complicating life for many birds that nest on the ground and have to fly from Africa to find sites with few predators (while) Warmer weather could bring predators north'. As climate changes, migratory birds or other endemic species may soon find themselves outnumbered by invasive ones.

Changes in seasonal temperatures and increases in global temperatures also affect the availability and proliferation of insects, which in turn are essential parts of the diets of many bird species. For instance, 'birds are sometimes hatching early in a warmer climate, but sometimes insect food can flourish even earlier. Pied Flycatcher birds in Europe for instance have suffered from a lack of caterpillars for their chicks.

Take, for instance, the critical endangered Siberian Crane, a wetland migratory bird whose numbers worldwide are down to 3000 individuals. The cranes breed in the Arctic confines of Russia and Siberia, and spend their winters in the mid or lower ranges of the Yangtze River. Unfortunately, this bird's Arctic tundra habitat is forecast to decline by 70 per cent. The tundra where they breed is not the only climate region on which the cranes rely on that is now in jeopardy, as a 'decreased precipitation, coupled with more intense rainfall events, also negatively affects the crane in its habitat in China'. Siberian Cranes have not been exempt to other climate changes, since 'increasing drought due to higher temperatures is thought to be one factor that caused a subpopulation of Siberian Crane, which once wintered in India's Keoladeo National Park, to shift out of the park and become locally extinct.

The Pied Flycatcher serves as another exam0ple of a bird species facing similar challenges. These long distance migratory birds are changing the timing of their migrations in an effort to adapt to climate change. The problem with this measure to keep up with climate change and its impact is that 'the plants and animals they interact with do not shift at the same rate'. In Europe, it has been observed that an earlier spring climax in insects numbers means that Pied Flycatchers no longer arrive from Africa in time to match food peaks with peak demands of their nestlings. The species has seen as a result a 90 percent decline in some of its European populations within the last two decades.

Other bird species have also seen their existence increasingly threatened in Australia. For instance, desertification and temperature increase are contributing to eliminate the habitat of many different species. For example, 'the habitat of the Golden Lowerbird is predicted to shrink by 97.5 per cent with a future warming at 3°C and a 10 per cent decline in rainfall', and an increase beyond 3°C would cause the bird to disappear entirely. Because, the Golden Lowerbird occupies the cooler areas in Australia more humid tropics in mountains enclosed by warmer regions, as temperatures rise, the habitat will continue to shrink.

In the United Kingdom, the North Sea saw an apian breeding collapse in the year 2004. the direct cause of this crash was a shortage of sandeels, a small fish essential to the diet of many birds, including the Hercules of all apian migrators, the Arctic Tern. This shortage of food was related to global warming, and according to the World Wildlife Fund Global Climate Change Programme, 'Warming ocean waters and major shifts in species that underpin the ocean food web are thought to be behind the major sandeel decline'.

The Arctic Terns (see Fig.2) demonstrate perfectly how susceptible migratory birds are to climate disruptions, especially since this is a bird whose annual journey round-trip totals between 22000 and 30000 miles. Since Arctic Terns live live upto 30 years, a single one of these 14-17 inches long, two-pound birds may travel during its lifetime more than 650000 miles. Interestingly enough, Arctic Terns see more daylight than any other creatures on the planet, 'since they are in both the Arctic and Antarctic during the periods of longest days.

Arctic Terns rely on the North Sea (see the map on Fig.7) as a source of food in their long journeys. In the year 2004, the terns saw their habitual feeding stop unable to supply them with enough food. In fact, 'no Arctic tern chicks were reared in the south of Shetland (archipelago in Northern Scotland in 2004. and although hundreds of Arctic Terns arrived at the RSPB's (a wild reserve owned by the Birdlife international, UK) Mousa reserve this spring, no young were fledged. All the large Arctic Tern colonies on Orkney (Northern

Scotland) failed and for the first time in living memory, none nested at the RSPB reserve on Papa Westray (also in Scotland)'. The Terns were not alone in their plight. The nearly 7000 pairs of Great Skuas in the Shetlands (another species dependent on the North Sea for food) produced only a handful of chicks and starving adult birds ate their own youngs.

The collapse of fish productivity in the North Sea in the year 2004 has been called by scientists, 'a regime shift', because 'rising sea temperatures have fundamentally changed the plankton mix to the detriment of sandeels'. The fishes that are essential as part of the diet of the many birds that stop in the North Sea to feed, as reported by Birdlife International in a press release entitled, "Seabirds in the North Sea : Victims of climate change?" Sandeels also are essential to other links of the marine food chain, which means that other fish and bird species have started to see their numbers drop as well, such as mackerels, cod, or kittiwakes (a seabird). The 2004 collapse was so severe that fishermen voluntarily shut down the fishery in the worst affect areas of the United Kingdom's North Sea. The Marine Policy Head of the Birdlife International concluded that 'we could be witnessing the single biggest change in the North Sea since it was formed 10000 years ago'.

So what ?

We know that bird species are great indicators of climate change - the canary in the coal mine - and as such, they are extremely vulnerable to all the impacts of global warming, particularly the species that depend on food sources on their specific stops along the way during their yearly migrations. We also know that a very significant percentage of these - one in eight bird species to be precise - are at risk due to warmer climate. But, why are bird species important in order to keep the ecosystems worldwide healthy?

If we can picture a world in which there is no seed dispersal, pollination or pest control naturally done, they we would be picturing a world devoid of bird species which do the planet an essential ecological service. In fact, studies done as to the cost of such services provided by nature to humanity (by insects, birds, plants) were estimated in a 1997 study to be 30 trillian dollars, according to Harvard University Professor Emeritus, E.O. Wilson (from the BBC Planet Earth series - Saving Species - fragment).

In the case of migratory birds, if we consider their stopping to feed and breed in particular regions in perfect timing with the massive hatching of worms, or any other insect, we have a natural pest and parasite control in these winged pilgrims. And, at the same time, these birds may be essential to nourish other creatures in the same ecosystem, essential predators at higher level of the food chain. The arrival of these birds to their breeding grounds, the eggs they produce and eventually their nestlings, are an essential source of food for small predators to feed on and to nourish their young. A disturbance in the population and arrival time of migratory birds would entail problems for all predators that await this annual food bonanza.

The problems faced by the bird populations worldwide, and especially by migratory birds that may be traveling upto te3ns of thousands of miles, mean that drastic changes in any single world region could push a wide variety of bird species out of existence. Human activity responsible for greenhouse emissions is eliminating at unprecedented rates all that too many species need to survive and to keep the ecosystems alive and healthy. Birds such as the Floreana Mockingbird (Nesomimus trifascialus) of the Galapagos Islands of Ecuador – now a critically endangered bird – is yet another casualty, among countless others. These birds live on two small islands, Champions and Gardner-by-Floreana and its total population is now fewer than 60 individuals.

Unfortunately, for all animal species the very few measures taken to counter global warming can actually be more damaging and make matters sores. The IUCN showed that 'in Papua New Guinea, increased cultivation of the pal oil – a source of biofuel – has accelerated deforestation. This, in turn, poses a new threat to bird species including the New Britain Goshawk'. In the words of Stuart Butchart of Birdlife International, 'Species are being hit by the double whammy of habitat loss and climate change, populations become fragmented, the effect of climate change can have an even greater impact, leading to an increased risk of local extinctions'. Sadly, within decades, the spectacular winged migrations.

❑❑❑

Appendices

Appendix I : List of Zoos in India

Zoos are primarily dry facilities where animals are confined within enclosures and displayed to the public, and in which they may also be bred. Such facilities include zoos, safari parks, animal theme parks, aviaries, butterfly zoos, and reptile centres, as well as wildlife sanctuaries and nature reserves, where visitors are allowed.

The Central Zoo Authority of India (CZA) is the Governing Authority of all zoos in India and is an associate member of the World Association of Zoos and Aquariums (WAZA).

Zoos in India

Nandankanan Zoological Park, Bhubaneshwar, Odisha

Assam State Zoo-cum-Botanical Garden, Guwahati, Assam

Allen Forest Zoo, Kanpur, Uttar Pradesh

Alipore Zoological Gardens, Kolkata, West Bengal

Aizawl Zoo, Aizawl, Mizoram

Amirthi Zoological Park, Vellore, Tamil Nadu

Arinagar Anna Zoological Park (Vandalur Zoo), Chennai, Tamil Nadu

Birsa Deer Park (Kalamati Birsa Mrig Vihar), Ranchi

Chattbir Zoo, Zirakpur, Punjab

Chennai Snake Park Trust, Chennai, Tamil Nadu

Indore Zoo, Indore, Madhya Pradesh

Indira Gandhi Zoological Park, Vishakhapatnam, Andhra Pradesh

Jawaharlal Nehru Biological Park, Bokaro Steel City, Jharkhand

Jaipur Zoo, Jaipur, Rajasthan

Gulab Bagh and Zoo, Udaipur, Rajasthan

Bennerghatta National Park, Bengaluru, Karnataka

Jheme Park, Jamshedpur, Jharkhand

Jijamata Udyaan, Mumbai, Maharashtra

Jhargram Zoo, Jhargram, West Bengal

Kankaria Zoo, Ahmedabad, Gujarat

Lucknow Zoo, Lucknow, Uttar Pradesh

Madras Crocodile Bank Trust, Chennai, Tamil Nadu

Marble Palace Zoo, Kolkata, West Bengal

Mysore Zoo, Mysore, Karnatak

National Zoological Park,Delhi

Nehru Zoological Park, Hyderabad, Telangana

Padmaja Naidu Himalayan Zoological Park, Darjeeling, West Bengal

Parassinikkadavu Snake Park, Chennai, Tamil Nadu

Ranchi Zoo (Bhagwan Birsa Munda Biological Park), Ranchi, Jharkhand

Sakkarbaug Zoological Garden, Junagadh, Gujarat

Tata Steel Zoological Park (Jubilee Park), Jamshedpur, Jharkhand

Sarthana Zoo, Surat, Gujarat

Sanjay Gandhi Jaivik Udyan, Patna, Bihar

Sipahijola Wildlife Sanctuary, Tripura

Sri venkateswara Zoological Park, Tirupati, Andhra Pradesh

Rajiv Gandhi Zoological Park, Pune, Maharashtra

Thiruvananthapuram zoo, Trivandrum, Kerala

Tilyar Zoo, Rohtak, Haryana

Pt. GB Pant High Altitude Zoo, Nainital, Uttrakhand

Appendix II : Wildlife Sanctuaries of India

Year	Name	State	Area(km²)
	Spike Island Wildlife Sanctuary	Andaman and Nicobar Islands	211.7
1985	Interview Island Wildlife Sancuary	Andaman and Nicobar Islands	133
1987	Landfall Island Wildlife Sanctuary	Andaman and Nicobar Islands	29.48
1987	Lohabarrack Salt Water crocodile Santuary	Andaman and Nicobar Islands	22.21
1987	Defence Island Wildlife Sanctuary	Andaman and Nicobar Islands	10.49
1987	Cinque Island Wildlife Sanctuary	Andaman and Nicobar Islands	9.51
1987	Flat Island Wildlife Sanctuary	Andaman and Nicobar Islands	9.36
1987	Buchaan Island	Andaman and Nicobar Islands	933
1987	Barren Island Wildlife Sanctuary	Andaman and Nicobar Islands	8.1
1987	Kyd Island	Andaman and Nicobar Islands	8
1987	Shearme Island	Andaman and Nicobar Islands	7.85
1987	Paget Island AN	Andaman and Nicobar Islands	7.36
1987	Tilanchang Island	Andaman and Nicobar Islands	6.83
1977	Narcondum Island	Andaman and Nicobar Islands	6.81
1987	West Island	Andaman and Nicobar Islands	6.4
1987	East Island	Andaman and Nicobar Islands	6.11
1987	Ranger Island	Andaman and Nicobar Islands	4.26
1987	Swamp Island	Andaman and Nicobar Islands	4.09

1987	East (Tingling) Island	Andaman and Nicobar Islands	3.55
1977	North Reef Island	Andaman and Nicobar Islands	3.48
1987	Bennet Island	Andaman and Nicobar Islands	3.46
1987	Talabatcha Island	Andaman and Nicobar Islands	3.21
1987	Point Island	Andaman and Nicobar Islands	3.07
1987	Bondoville Island	Andaman and Nicobar Islands	2.55
1987	Table (Delgarno) Island	Andaman and Nicobar Islands	2.29
1985	Battimalve Island	Andaman and Nicobar Islands	3.29
1987	James Island	Andaman and Nicobar Islands	2.1
1987	Reef Island	Andaman and Nicobar Islands	1.74
1987	Table (Excelsior) Island	Andaman and Nicobar Islands	1.69
1977	South Sentinel Island	Andaman and Nicobar Islands	1.61
1987	Sandy Island	Andaman and Nicobar Islands	1.58
1987	Roper Island	Andaman and Nicobar Islands	1.46
1987	Pitman Island	Andaman and Nicobar Islands	1.37
1987	South Brother Island	Andaman and Nicobar Islands	1.24
1987	South Brother Island	Andaman and Nicobar Islands	1.24
1987	South Reef Island	Andaman and Nicobar Islands	1.17
1987	Bluff Island	Andaman and Nicobar Islands	1.14

1987	Sir Huge Rose Island	Andaman and Nicobar Islands	1.06
1987	Tample Island	Andaman and Nicobar Islands	1.04
1987	Ross Island	Andaman and Nicobar Islands	1.01
1970	Nalapattu Bird Sanctuary	Andhra Pradesh	4040
1978	Nagarjunsagar-Srisailam Tiger Reserve	Andhra Pradesh & Telangana	3568
ND	Gundla Brahmeshwarm Wildlife Sanctuary	Andhra Pradesh	1194
1963	Kolleru Lake	Andhra Pradesh	673
ND	Rollapadu Wildlife Sanctuary	Andhra Pradesh	614
1978	Popikonda Wildlife Sanctuary	Andhra Pradesh	591
1989	Sri Venkateswara National Park	Andhra Pradesh	353
1976	Pulicat Lake Bird Sanctuary	Andhra Pradesh	327.33
ND	Sri Lankamalleswara Wildlife Sanctuary	Andhra Pradesh	464.42
ND	Koundinya Wildlife Sanctuary	Andhra Pradesh	357
1978	Coringa Wildlife Sanctuary	Andhra Pradesh	235.79
ND	Krishna Wildlife Sanctuary	Andhra Pradesh	194.81
1972	Kambalakonda Wildlife Sanctuary	Andhra Pradesh	71
ND	Lanjamadugu Wildlife Sanctuary	Andhra Pradesh	ND
1977	Pakhuri Tiger Reserve	Arunachal Pradesh	861.95
1991	Dibang	Arunachal Pradesh	41.49
1989	Kamland	Arunachal Pradesh	783
1980	Mehao	Arunachal Pradesh	281.5
1989	Eagleneet Wildlife Sanctuary	Arunachal Pradesh	217
1978	D'ering Memorial Wildlife Sanctuary	Arunachal Pradesh	190
1978	Itanagar Wildlife Sanctuary	Arunachal Pradesh	140.3
1989	Seesa Orchid Sanctuary	Arunachal Pradesh	100
1991	Kane Wildlife Sanctuary	Arunachal Pradesh	55
ND	Talley Valley Wildlife Sanctuary	Arunachal Pradesh	337
1905	Kaziranga National Park	Assam	430

1980	Bornadi Wildlife Sanctuary	Assam	26.22
1989	Bipor Bil	Assam	40
ND	Garampani Wildlife Sanctuary	Assam	6.05
1997	Hoollongapur Gibbon Sanctuary	Assam	2098.62
1928	Manas National Park	Assam	391
1934	Sonal Rupai Wildlife Sanctuary	Assam	175
1985	Nameri National Park	Assam	137.07
1985	Orang National Park	Assam	72.6
1979	Laokhowa Wildlife Sanctuary	Assam	70.14
ND	Pabha Wildlife Sanctuary	Assam	49
1987	Pobitora Wildlife Sanctuary	Assam	38.83
1978	Kaimur Wildlife Sanctuary	Bihar	1342.22
1976	Bhimband Wildlife Sanctuary	Bihar	681.9
1978	Balmikinagar Wildlife Sanctuary	Bihar	461.6
1976	Gautam Buddha Wildlife Sanctuary	Bihar	259.6
1978	Lawalang	Bihar	211.03
1985	Nakti Dam	Bihar	206.4
1986	Kabar	Bihar	204
1976	Mahuadaur	Bihar	63.25
1984	Parasnath	Bihar	49.23
1978	Rajgir	Bihar	35.84
ND	Topchandhi	Bihar	ND
ND	Sukhna	Chandigarh	25.42
1975	Achanakmar Wildlife Sanctuary	Chhattisgarh	577.55
1983	Bhairamgarh Wildlife sanctuary	Chhattisgarh	138.95
1976	Baranawapara Wildlife Sanctuary	Chhattisgarh	244.66
1972	Udanti Wildlife Sanctuary	Chhattisgarh	232
1978	Semarsot Wildlife Sanctuary	Chhattisgarh	430.36
1974	Sitanadi Wildlife Sanctuary	Chhattisgarh	556
1978	Tamor Pingla Wildlife Sanctuary	Chhattisgarh	608.55
1983	Pamed Wildlife Sanctuary	Chhattisgarh	262
1983	Bhairamgarh Wildlife Sanctuary	Chhattisgarh	138.95
1975	Badalkohl Wildlife Sanctuary	Chhattisgarh	104.35

1975	Achanakamar	Chhattisgarh	551.55
1972	Gomarda Reserve Forest	Chhattisgarh	277.82
ND	Indra Prayadarshini	Delhi	13.2
1967	Bhagwan Mahavir	Goa	148.52
1968	Bhagwan Mahavir	Goa	105
1972	Bondla Wildlife Sanctuary	Goa	8
1979	Salim Ali Bird Sanctuary	Goa	1.8
1982	Spoolpaneshwar Wildlife Sanctuary	Gujarat	607.7
1989	Balaram -Ambaji Wildlife Sanctuary	Gujarat	542.08
1986	Kutch Desert Wildlife Sanctuary	Gujarat	7506.22
1973	Indian Wild Ass Sanctuary	Gujarat	4953.7
1965	Gir Forest National Park	Gujarat	1153.42
1981	Narayan Sarovar Sanctuary	Gujarat	765.79
1980	Marine National Park, Gulf of Kutch	Gujarat	293.03
1979	Barda Wildlife Sanctuary	Gujarat	192.31
1978	Jessore	Gujarat	180.66
1990	Purna	Gujarat	160.84
1990	Jambughoda	Gujarat	130.38
1969	Nal Sarovar	Gujarat	120.82
1982	Ratanmahal	Gujarat	55.65
1989	Paniya	Gujarat	39.69
1988	Rampura	Gujarat	15.01
ND	Khijadiya	Gujarat	ND
ND	Dhumkhal	Gujarat	ND
1988	Thor Bird Sanctuary	Gujarat	153
1987	Chautala	Haryana	113.96
1978	Bir Shikargarh	Haryana	10.93
1982	Rupa Bhabha Sanctuary	Himachal Pradesh	354.14
1962	Seehu Tuan Nala wildlife Sanctuary	Himachal Pradesh	655.32
1962	Tundah wildlife Sanctuary	Himachal Pradesh	419.48
1962	Kugti wildlife Sanctuary	Himachal Pradesh	330
1983	Pong Dam Sanctuary	Himachal Pradesh	322.7

1962	Nagru Dam Sanctuary	Himachal Pradesh	243.13
1962	Bandli	Himachal Pradesh	239.47
1962	Govind Sagar and Naina Devi	Himachal Pradesh	120.67
1976	Chail	Himachal Pradesh	110.04
1949	Gamgul Siahbehi	Himachal Pradesh	105.46
1962	Darlaghat	Himachal Pradesh	98.71
1962	Shikari Devi	Himachal Pradesh	71.19
1976	Tirthan	Himachal Pradesh	68.25
1954	Kanawar	Himachal Pradesh	61.57
1985	Churdhar	Himachal Pradesh	56.59
1962	Raksham Chitkul	Himachal Pradesh	38.27
1962	Naina Devi	Himachal Pradesh	37.19
1962	Talra	Himachal Pradesh	36.16
1962	Majathal	Himachal Pradesh	31.64
1964	Manali Sanctuary	Himachal Pradesh	31.27
1949	Kalatop and Khajjiar	Himachal Pradesh	30.69
1962	Lippa Asrang	Himachal Pradesh	29.53
1962	Daranghati	Himachal Pradesh	27.01
1954	Khokhan	Himachal Pradesh	17.6
1958	Simbalbara	Himachal Pradesh	17.2
1954	Kais	Himachal Pradesh	12.2
ND	Ranuka	Himachal Pradesh	ND
ND	Shilli	Himachal Pradesh	ND
ND	Karakoram Wildlife Sanctuary	Jammu & Kashmir	1800
1987	Lachipora	Jammu & Kashmir	800
1987	Overa-Aru	Jammu & Kashmir	425
1988	Kanji Wildlife Sanctuary	Jammu & Kashmir	250
1987	Gulmarg	Jammu & Kashmir	186
1987	Hirpora Wildlife Sanctuary	Jammu & Kashmir	341
1981	Surinsar-Mansar	Jammu & Kashmir	39.58
1981	Nandini	Jammu & Kashmir	33.72
2008	Achabal	Jammu & Kashmir	ND
1987	Limber	Jammu & Kashmir	26
ND	Tongri	Jammu & Kashmir	20
1981	Ramnagar	Jammu & Kashmir	12.09

ND	Hokarsar	Jammu & Kashmir	10
1987	Baltal	Jammu & Kashmir	3
1987	Changtang Wildlife Sanctuary	Jammu & Kashmir	4000
1976	Palamau Tiger Reserve	Jharkhand	767
1976	Dalma Wildlife Sanctuary	Jharkhand	193.22
1977	Hazaribagh	Jharkhand	186.25
1985	Koderma	Jharkhand	177.95
1974	Mookambika Wildlife Sanctuary	Karnataka	247
1974	Melkote Temple	Karnataka	49.82
1974	Nugu Wildlife Sanctuary	Karnataka	30.32
1974	Ghataprpabha Bird Sanctuary	Karnataka	29.78
1985	Arabithittu Wildlife Sanctuary	Karnataka	13.5
1985	Adichuhhchanagiri Wildlife Sanctuary	Karnataka	0.88
1974	Bharda Wildlife Sanctuary	Karnataka	492.46
2011	Bhimgad Wildlife Sanctuary	Karnataka	190.42
1987	Biligiriranga Swamy Temple Wildlife Sanctuary	Karnataka	539.58
1974	Brahmagiri Wildlife Sanctuary	Karnataka	181.29
1987	Cauvery Wildlife Sanctuary	Karnataka	510.16
ND	Dandeli Wildlife Sanctuary	Karnataka	834.16
ND	Gudavi Bird Sanctuary	Karnataka	0.74
ND	Mandagadde Bird Sanctuary	Karnataka	0.005
ND	Melukote Temple Wildlife Sanctuary	Karnataka	45.82
1987	Pushpagiri Wildlife Sanctuary	Karnataka	102.59
ND	Ranganthittu	Karnataka	0.67
1974	Ranibernur Blackbuck Sanctuary	Karnataka	119
1972	Sharavathi Valley Wildlife Sanctuary	Karnataka	413.23
1974	Shettihalli Wildlife Sanctuary	Karnataka	395.6
1974	Someshwara Wildlife Sanctuary	Karnataka	88.4
1987	Talakaveri Wildlife Sanctuary	Karnataka	105
1950	Periyar National Park	Kerala	472
1973	Waynad	Kerala	344.44

1973	Parambikulam Wildlife Sanctuary	Kerala	285
1958	Neyyar	Kerala	128
1958	Peechi-Vazhani Wildlife Sanctuary	Kerala	125
1984	Chimmony Wildlife Sanctuary	Kerala	105
1984	Shenduruny	Kerala	100.32
1984	Chinnar	Kerala	90.44
1976	Idukki	Kerala	77
1984	Aralam	Kerala	55
1983	Peppara	Kerala	53
1983	Thattekkad Bird Sanctuary	Kerala	25
ND	Kumarakom	Kerala	ND
2010	Malabar Wildlife Sanctuary	Kerala	74.21
1977	Bori Wildlife Sanctuary	Madhya Pradesh	518.25
1978	Bagdara Wildlife Sanctuary	Madhya Pradesh	478.90
1983	Phen Sanctuary	Madhya Pradesh	110.24
1981	Ghatigaon Sanctuary	Madhya Pradesh	512
1974	Gandhi Sagar Sanctuary	Madhya Pradesh	368.62
1981	Kaqera Wildlife Sanctuary	Madhya Pradesh	202.21
1981	Ken Ghariyal Sanctuary	Madhya Pradesh	45
1955	Kheoni Sanctuary	Madhya Pradesh	134.78
1974	Narsinghgarh Wildlife Sanctuary	Madhya Pradesh	57.19
1978	National Chambal Sanctuary	Madhya Pradesh	320
1975	Nauradehi Wildlife Sanctuary	Madhya Pradesh	1034.52
1977	Pachmarhi Sanctuary	Madhya Pradesh	461.85
1983	Panpatha Wildlife Sanctuary	Madhya Pradesh	245.84
1981	Kuno Wildlife Sanctuary	Madhya Pradesh	344.68
1976	Ratapaik Tiger Reserve	Madhya Pradesh	688.79
1975	Sanjay-Durbi Wildlife Sanctuary	Madhya Pradesh	364.69
1976	Singhori Wildlife Sanctuary	Madhya Pradesh	287.91
1981	Son Ghariyal Sanctuary	Madhya Pradesh	41.8
1983	Sardarpur Sanctuary	Madhya Pradesh	348.12
1985	Melghat	Maharashtra	597.23
1986	Tadoma Andhari Tiger Project	Maharashtra	625.4

1985	Koyna Wildlife Sanctuary	Maharashtra	423.55
1958	Radhanagri Wildlife Sanctuary	Maharashtra	371.88
1986	Kalsubai Harishchandra	Maharashtra	361.71
1986	Jaikwadi	Maharashtra	341.05
1986	Painganga	Maharashtra	324.62
1979	Great Indian Burstard Sanctuary	Maharashtra	8496.44
1985	Chandoli National Park	Maharashtra	308.97
1986	Gautala Autramghat Sanctuar	Maharashtra	260.61
1969	Yawat	Maharashtra	177.52
1970	Magzira	Maharashtra	152.81
1986	Chaprala	Maharashtra	134.78
1985	Bhimashankar	Maharashtra	130.78
1986	Nandpur Madmeshwar	Maharashtra	100.12
1986	Aner Da	Maharashtra	82.94
1988	Katepurna	Maharashtra	73.69
1986	Phansad Wildlife Sanctuary	Maharashtra	69.79
1970	Bor	Maharashtra	61.1
1970	Tansa	Maharashtra	30.41
1987	Malvan Marine	Maharashtra	29.12
1985	Sagershwar	Maharashtra	10.87
ND	Dhakna Kolkaz	Maharashtra	ND
ND	Gandhari	Maharashtra	ND
ND	Yedshi Ramling Ghat	Maharashtra	22.37
ND	Wainganga	Maharashtra	ND
1989	Yagoupokpi Lokchao	Manipur	184.8
1981	Nongkhyllem	Meghalaya	29
ND	Bhagmara	Meghalaya	ND
ND	Siju	Meghalaya	ND
1985	Dampa Tiger Reserve	Mizoram	550
1991	Khawnglung	Mizoram	41
1991	Ngenpui	Mizoram	150
ND	Fakim	Nagaland	ND
1975	Itanki	Nagaland	202.02
ND	Pulebatze	Nagaland	ND
1988	Badrama Sanctuary	Odisha	304.03

1981	Baisipalli Wildlife Sanctuary	Odisha	168.35
1984	Balukhand Konark	Odisha	71.72
1975	Bhitarkanika	Odisha	70
1982	Chandaka Dampara	Odisha	175.79
1987	Chilka Bird Sanctuary	Odisha	1100
1987	Nalbana Bird Sanctuary	Odisha	1100
1985	Debrigarh wildlife Sanctuary	Odisha	346.91
1978	Hadgarh	Odisha	191.06
1991	Karlapat	Odisha	147.06
1981	Kotgarh	Odisha	399.05
1984	Kuldiha wildlife Sanctuary	Odisha	300
1985	Lakhari Valley	Odisha	185.87
1982	Khalasuni	Odisha	116
1976	Satkosia Gorge Wildlife Sanctuary	Odisha	795.52
1979	Simlipal National Park	Odisha	845.7
1986	Sunabeda Wildlife Sanctuary	Odisha	600
ND	Ushakothi	Odisha	ND
ND	Bir Motibagh	Punjab	ND
1975	Abohar	Punjab	188.24
ND	Bir Bunnerheri	Punjab	ND
ND	Bir Gurdialpura	Punjab	ND
1982	Harike Lake	Punjab	43
1960	Mount Abu Wildlife Sanctuary	Rajasthan	288.84
1985	Baretha	Rajasthan	192.76
ND	Bassi	Rajasthan	ND
1983	Bhensrodagarh	Rajasthan	229.14
1983	Chambal	Rajasthan	280
1955	Darrah Wildlife Sanctuary	Rajasthan	ND
ND	Garhial	Rajasthan	ND
1956	Jaisamand	Rajasthan	52
1955	Jaswant Sagar Wildlife Sanctuary	Rajasthan	ND
1980	Jawahar Sagar	Rajasthan	100
1983	keladevi Wildlife Sanctuary	Rajasthan	676
1971	Kumbhalgarh	Rajasthan	578.26

1980	Nahargarh	Rajasthan	50
1983	Pulwari Wildlife Sanctuary	Rajasthan	511.41
1982	Jamwa Ramgarh Wildlife Sanctuary	Rajasthan	300
1982	Ramgarh Vishdhari Wildlife Sanctuary	Rajasthan	307
1955	Sariska Tiger Reserve	Rajasthan	866
1984	Sawai Mansingh	Rajasthan	103.25
1983	Shergarh	Rajasthan	98.71
1979	Sita Mata Wildlife Sanctuary	Rajasthan	422.94
ND	Sundha Mata	Rajasthan	107
ND	Tal Chhapar Sanctuary	Rajasthan	ND
1983	Todgarh Rawali Wildlife Sanctuary	Rajasthan	495.26
1955	Van Vihar	Rajasthan	59.93
1984	Varsey Rhododendron Sanctuary	Sikkim	51.76
1984	Farmbong Lho	Sikkim	51.76
1984	Pangolakha Wildlife Sanctuary	Sikkim	ND
1987	Meanam	Sikkim	35.34
1984	Shingba Rhododendron	Sikkim	32.25
1988	Kalakkade Mundanthurai Tiger Reserve	Tamil Nadu	895
ND	Kalakkadu	Tamil Nadu	223.58
ND	Karikili	Tamil Nadu	ND
ND	Mudumalai National Park	Tamil Nadu	321.55
ND	Mukkurthi	Tamil Nadu	78.46
ND	Point Calimere	Tamil Nadu	17.26
ND	Pulicat Lake Bird Sanctuary	Tamil Nadu	153.67
2008	Sathyamangalam Wildlife Sanctuary	Tamil Nadu	1411.6
ND	Shenbagathoppu Grizzled Squirrel Wildlife Sanctuary	Tamil Nadu	480
ND	Vallanadu	Tamil Nadu	16.41
ND	Vedantangal	Tamil Nadu	0.3
ND	Vettamngudi	Tamil Nadu	ND

1953	Eturnagaram Wildlife Sanctuary	Telangana	803
1965	Kawal Wildlife Sanctuary	Telangana	893
1977	Kinnerasani Wildlife Sanctuary	Telangana	655.41
1978	Manjira Wildlife Sanctuary	Telangana	20
1952	Pakhal Wildlife Sanctuary	Telangana	879.3
1952	Pocharam Forest & Wildlife Sanctuary	Telangana	130
1980	Pranahita Wildlife Sanctuary	Telangana	136.02
1978	Shivaram Wildlife Sanctuary	Telangana	36.29
1988	Gumti Wildlife Sanctuary	Tripura	ND
1987	Sepahijala	Tripura	389.54
1987	Trishna	Tripura	170.56
ND	Asan Bradge Bird Watching	Uttar Pradesh	ND
1957	Chandra Prabha Sanctuary	Uttar Pradesh	78
ND	Chilla	Uttar Pradesh	ND
1982	Kaimoor Sanctuary	Uttar Pradesh	500.75
1976	Katarniaghat Wildlife Sanctuary	Uttar Pradesh	400
1977	Ranipur Sanctuary	Uttar Pradesh	230.31
1987	Sohabi Barwal Sanctuary	Uttar Pradesh	428.02
1986	Hastinapur Sanctuary	Uttar Pradesh	2073
ND	Mahavir Swamy	Uttar Pradesh	ND
ND	Nawabganj	Uttar Pradesh	ND
ND	Samaspur	Uttar Pradesh	ND
1989	Okhla Bird Sanctuary	Uttar Pradesh	4.00
1990	Sandi Bird Sanctuary	Uttar Pradesh	3.09
1979	National Chambal Sanctuary	Uttar Pradesh	635
1986	Ascot Musk Deer Sanctuary	Uttrakhand	599.93
1988	Binsar	Uttrakhand	45.59
1954	Govind Pashu Vihar Wildlife Sanctuary	Uttrakhand	481.04
1972	Kedarnath Wildlife Sanctuary	Uttrakhand	975.24
1987	Sonandi Wildlife Sanctuary	Uttrakhand	301.18
1976	Singlalila National Park	West Bengal	362.4
1986	Buxa Tiger Reserve	West Bengal	251.89
1976	Murti Wildlife	West Bengal	127.22

1976	Senchal	West Bengal	38.88
1976	Lothian Island	West Bengal	38
1976	Holiday Island	West Bengal	5.95
ND	Bibhutibhushan	West Bengal	ND
ND	Bethudahari	West Bengal	ND
ND	Ballabhpur	West Bengal	ND
ND	Chapramari	West Bengal	ND
ND	Gorumara	West Bengal	ND
ND	Jore Pokhri	West Bengal	ND
1959	Mahananda	West Bengal	159
ND	Parnadhan	West Bengal	ND
ND	Ramnabagan	West Bengal	ND
ND	Raiganj	West Bengal	ND

Appendix III : List of Ramsar (Wetland) Sites in India

S.No.	Name	Location	Designated	Area (km^2)
1.	Ashtamudi Wetland	Kerala	19.8.02	614
2.	Bhitarkanika Mangroves	Orisha	19.8.02	650
3.	Bhoj Wetland	Madhya Pradesh	19.8.02	32
4.	Chandra Taal	Himachal Pradesh	8.11.05	49
5.	Chilika Lake	Orissa	1.1.81	1165
6.	Deepor Beel	Assam	19.8.02	40
7.	East Calcutta Wetlands	West Bengal	19.8.02	125
8.	Harike Wetland	Punjab	23.3.90	41
9.	Hokersar Wetland	Jammu & Kashmir	8.11.05	13.75
10.	Kanjli Wetland	Punjab	22.1.02	1.83
11.	Keoladeo National Park	Rajasthan	1.10.81	28.73
12.	Kolleru Lake	Andhra Pradesh	19.8.02	901
13.	Loktak Lake	Manipur	23.03.90	266
14.	Nalsarovar Bird Sanctuary	Gujarat	24.9.12	123
15.	Point Calimere Wildlife and Bird Sanctuary	Tamil Nadu	19.8.02	385
16.	Pong Dam Lake	Himachal Pradesh	19.8.02	156.62
17.	Renuka Wetland	Himachal Pradesh	8.11.05	2
18.	Ropar	Punjab	22.1.02	13.65
19.	Rudrasagar Lake	Tripura	8.11.05	2.4
20.	Sambhar Lake	Rajasthan	23.3.90	240
21.	Sasthamkotta Lake	Kerala	19.8.02	3.73
22.	Surinsar-Mansar Lakes	Jammu & Kashmir	8.11.05	3.5
23.	Tsomoriri	Jammu & Kashmir	19.8.02	120

24.	Upper Ganga River (Brijghat to Narora Stretch)	Uttar Pradesh	8.11.05	265.9
25.	Vembanad-Kol Wetland	Kerala	19.8.02	1512.5
26.	Wular Lake	Jammu and Kashmir	23.3.90	189

❑❑❑